EAT TODAY TO THINK TOMORROW!

J. I. Rodale, one of America's outstanding proponents of natural foods, gives you his controversial plan for eating your way to improved mental health and increased mental vitality.

According to Mr. Rodale, Vitamin B complex helps the brain maintain a sound mental balance. Here he gives the results of his research on what foods and food supplements offer the richest supply of these essential vitamins, and discusses the "brain-sharpening" possibilities of Vitamins A and C, and the still-mysterious role Vitamin E may play in nutrition.

Vitamins—plus proteins and exercise—are a beginning. Find out all about the unorthodox Rodale system, and the wonders it might perform for you.

This book might help you to
EAT BETTER • THINK BETTER • BE BETTER

RODALE'S SYSTEM FOR MENTAL POWER AND NATURAL HEALTH

J. I. RODALE

PYRAMID BOOKS • NEW YORK

**RODALE'S SYSTEM FOR
MENTAL POWER AND NATURAL HEALTH**

A PYRAMID BOOK
Published by arrangement with Rodale Press, Inc.

Pyramid edition published June 1968
   Second printing, March 1969
   Third printing, July 1970
   Fourth printing, April 1971

Library of Congress Catalog Card Number: 66-13188

PYRAMID BOOKS are published by Pyramid Publications
A Division of The Walter Reade Organization, Inc.
444 Madison Avenue, New York, New York 10022, U.S.A.

Contents

Foreword

It is an accepted fact that good nutrition is required for good physical health. Athletes dine at special training tables and the diets of our astronauts are carefully selected. However, not too much thought has been given to the effect of diet on the thinking processes of people.

It may seem strange that I, a state senator and lawyer, am writing a preface to a book of this type. The orthodox approach would be a few complimentary paragraphs from a friendly medical doctor. But what Mr. Rodale says about diet and mental alertness goes to the heart of every day living, and in my observation through the years had his advice been followed in past years, we would be living in a better world today. Mr. Rodale cites convincing material that statesmen, industrialists, union organizers, educators, yes, even politicians, would do well to at least try what he prescribes. Perhaps we would have no wars, less poverty, better labor relations, improved education and better laws.

As chairman of the New York State Joint Legislative Committee on Motor Vehicles, Traffic and Highway Safety, I am deeply concerned about the soaring death rate on the highways of my state and the nation. I believe Mr. Rodale is on the right track in pointing out that the ability to make a quick emergency decision at the wheel may depend on the state of the driver's mental energy. To back up this theory, he cites an interesting study in which a group of truck drivers who took vitamin pills during a test period had fewer accidents than drivers of the same company who did not take the vitamins.

Mr. Rodale is not a food faddist. His very nature and his background makes him a realist. He was raised on the crowded east side of New York where he quickly learned the realities of life. Without a college education he became a selfmade man, chalking up successes in such unrelated fields as manufacturing, magazine publishing and writing.

I first met Mr. Rodale 35 years ago, but our interests in health matters have run parallel through the years. Mr. Rodale followed closely my bill in the 1965 New York Legislature—a first in the nation—which called for a warning label on every package of cigarettes sold in the State. He also has expressed keen interest in my legislative work to curb air pollution.

While setting a few guidelines to mental alertness, Mr. Rodale also preaches what has been passed on to us from biblical times—that we should eat in moderation. He disapproves of tobacco, but this is hardly the stand of a faddist in view of the substantial medical evidence linking cancer with cigarette smoking. He urges that drinking of alcohol be kept at a minimum, but he does not disapprove for he says "a drink once in a while on a social occasion, provided there are not too many social occasions," is O.K.

Mr. Rodale has only one ax to grind. That is, by following the principles laid down in this book there will be a great improvement in your mental capacity and ability and as a bonus, you will live longer.

SIMON J. LIEBOWITZ
State Senator from the 18th Senatorial District and the 38th Assembly District, New York

How You Will Benefit From This Book

MY PURPOSE in writing this book is to show people how to become more vital physically and more mentally alert. There is a potential as far as mental energy is concerned but it is definitely known that the average person develops and uses only about one-tenth of this power. There are too many persons who become physically fatigued, who get sick too often, whose work is of drab quality when suffering their chronic colds or headaches. Too much time is wasted at the dentist. It is possible to get more physical energy, to do away with headaches and dental cavities, to become much healthier generally. Methods and ideas will be discussed in this book to show how to obtain optimum mental health.

But the greater portion of this book will deal with methods to increase the store of one's mental energy. One sees about one too much mediocrity in thinking ability. Two persons may be similarly equipped in brain power, but one of them, for some reason utilizes his power more. It is the purpose of this book to try and find out why this is so.

Merely getting a college degree, reading books, or memorizing a lot of facts may not do it. To make intelligent decisions requires mental energy . . . the ability to cudgel the brain, to think deeply. Some persons remain on the surface . . . rarely penetrating deep enough into a question or problem to do anything with it.

What is needed is an ability to make the mind jump into quick action, plus the power to keep it on the *qui vive* until the thought has been completed and the decision made.

Why do some people have no difficulty in piling up ideas, while others hardly ever do so? There are ideas continually floating around about us, but the grade B mind does not have enough mental energy to grab hold of them.

11

The B person sees a thing—a word, a fact, a possibility, thinks about it vaguely . . . there is a little stir in his gray matter, momentarily. He wonders whether he should remember it, but quickly his mental energy dissipates . . . already he has forgotten the thing or word or possibility. It has vanished completely!

But your grade A mind pounces on such a thing and quickly turns it over 6 different ways. He gets hold of its tail, and keeps hold of it. He thinks about it long enough for it to make an indelible impression in his gray matter, or whatever it is that holds these impressions.

Social Dexterity Is Not Mental Ability

Now there are people who give a general impression of being highly intelligent. They are quick to give an answer of some kind, as long as it sounds like an answer. But whether it is right or wrong is not important to them, as long as they deliver it in a manner that *indicates* it is right. Some of them become college professors by memorizing the necessary factual material. Some of them who have a distinguished appearance and an eloquent method of speaking become college presidents. Many of these persons are what I call socially dexterous. They are the kind of people who get on committees, in fact who are prone to head committees . . . but who sow confusion, who bungle things up with their fancy rhetoric, and who destroy by compromising.

On the other hand there are uneducated, illiterate persons, who have high rates of mental energy and ability, who are extremely intelligent . . . like the Greek junk dealer who filed an income tax return with an annual income of a quarter of a million dollars, but who could sign his name only with an X. What could there be in the make-up of this Greek that sets him apart from some of our college professors?

A Remarkable Example

About 5 years ago, along with many other businessmen (I am also the owner of an electric manufacturing plant, employing about 400 persons), I visited a large General Electric factory at Louisville, Kentucky, to be shown some new developments in automation. I was amazed to see that the entire division, comprising over 10,000 workers, was under the management of a young man, not over 30 years old. And to watch him during the 2 days I was there was a revelation. What mental brilliance! He completely dominated the 60 grizzled businessmen who sat at his feet, listening to him talk to us after each section visit.

My theory was that such a thing just doesn't come out of the air. There is always a cause, as Voltaire has so aptly said. In a great many cases I believe it is in the person's nutrition. We are what we eat. A physician has said, what we eat today walks about tomorrow. Could it also be that what we eat today *"thinks"* tomorrow?

At the end of the second day I sought out this young man and questioned him about his diet. His reply was exactly what I had guessed. His preference since childhood had been for food high in animal protein, low in carbohydrates. He had always shunned sugarized foods, and bypassed the usual refined, sweet desserts. Of course there must have been other factors responsible for his mental ability—his environment, boyhood associates, the kind of conversation he was exposed to at the family table, etc. But I am sure that when a good diet is added to this, it can help.

I went away a wiser man both in the art of automation . . . the effect of man on the machine . . . and the effect of food on the human machine. Is it possible that our Greek friend also had a better diet, in the land where he came from, where the food is not so fragmentized as in our country, where the effect of the machine on our food, as devitalized it, eliminating from it essential fractions because they interfere with the smooth operation of the food as it goes through the processing machinery?

But the brain needs these missing parts. It must be nourished with wholeness! We must make sure that the bloodstream feeds the necessary minerals and vitamins into the network of nerves, blood-vessels and tissues of which the brain is composed. From the research I have done, and it consists of studying hundreds of medical researches performed in conservative medical and other institutions, I find that there is a very direct connection between what one eats, and how the mind functions.

Dr. George Gallup's Idea

Dr. George Gallup has just written a book called *The Miracle Ahead* (Harper and Row), in which he says that nobody is very good at thinking. He learned this from years of polling the thoughts of others. He says that not only do individuals fail in their power of thinking, but that this also applies to institutions formed for making group decisions. Of course "Nobody" is a rather all-inclusive word. I would have said that painfully few people know how to think.

Dr. Gallup's idea to teach people how to think is to revise our educational system. He advises a "new methodology" in which surveys, statistics and computers will be the chief tools. In my opinion he is overlooking the basic symptom or cause of our mass mental inertia—malnutrition. In my opinion all the surveys and statistics and computers in the world will not give a poorly nourished individual the power to think nimbly and with a good degree of intelligence . . . this book will tell you why.

Are You Depending on Nature?

If you don't have a plan, then you will be perhaps one out of a thousand who somehow naturally seems to be mentally endowed. If you think you can become brilliant by merely eating the so-called balanced diet and that that is nature's plan, then you may be left out in the cold about ever becoming a number one brain. Nature is interested in one thing, and one thing only, and that is the perpetuation of the species. Everything in nature, the plants, the animals, the elements are part of a scheme of reproduction of the species, to perpetuate the race, and no doubt through the process of evolution nature has found that her plan will operate better without the help of any human geniuses, because as soon as a genius appears (and this is always by some accident of nature) he usually considers himself smarter than nature and begins to figure out ways to make life easier, whereas nature wants life to be harder. A life of ease weakens the human body, which contributes to impotence and to the eventual disappearance of man from the face of the earth!

To nature, a genius is a freak or a maverick . . . comes a Napoleon and millions have to die . . . which alarms nature . . . comes a Priestley and oxygen is discovered and today some people are getting sick from overdoses of artificial oxygen. . . . In nature's plan she doesn't give a rap whether we know that there is such a thing as oxygen. According to nature, we can continue to reproduce without being aware that oxygen is necessary to activate body processes. Nature says, "You want oxygen? Then get out into the air!" But civilized man is now figuring how to stay indoors by placing huge plastic "bubbles" over vast outdoor areas. He knows about oxygen but from his acts you would think he doesn't!

You Need More Than a "Balanced" Diet

The point I wish to make is this: if you eat the ordinary, even the balanced diet, that nature makes available to you, you can only expect to be a normal average individual—far from a genius! And this is the kind of diet that the medical profession recommends for you. But if you study this book carefully, you will finally agree that nature has left herself vulnerable—she did not foresee that man would some day learn to extract the most potent nutrition from her foods—the vitamins, and by taking large amounts of these vitamin substances to become much healthier than even nature intended, and much more intelligent, for health and intelligence go together.

So, it is not impossible to expect that in the foreseeable future, scientists will learn much more about vitamins and their effect on the human brain, and thus raise the level of human intelligence a hundredfold, so that there will be thousands of geniuses and near-geniuses.

By that time man will have learned how to use such intelligence without becoming so scientific that that very scientificalness would be our destruction. And you who are reading this book should understand that you can remove yourself from nature's pool of averageness. Don't let nature push you around.

We can do it through our diet. Food can create miracles! The bees will completely change the character and physical abilities of a drone bee, by feeding it with royal jelly. In this manner they will produce a queen bee. Paul de Kruif has written about interesting changes in animals on super-charged diets. Then why not people? In man's literature he has speculated on this subject, but always from his pessimistic imagination he creates monstrous Dybbuks and Frankensteins. He turns Jekylls into Hydes, but he doesn't seem to want to lift his head up and create angels.

The Politicians and the Bees

We can do it! We can start with our politicians, statesmen, industrialists, union organizers, educators, and so forth. By feeding them according to the principles laid down in this book, we might transform them into a new type of individual who will give us higher types of government, business, education, and so forth. How unscientific it is, in an era of modern science and technology to permit wages to be determined by methods of open warfare. Something is physically and mentally wrong with the leaders of capital and labor, when they permit such a state of affairs to continue to exist.

The late Dr. Raymond Pearl of Johns Hopkins University in his famous book, *The Biology of Death,* has this to say: "Attempts at social control of the germ-plasm—the innate inherited constitutional make-up of a people, by eugenic 'legislation,' have not been conspicuously successful. . . . As an animal breeder of some years' experience, I have no doubt whatever that almost any breeder of average intelligence, if given omnipotent control over the activities of human beings, could, in a few generations, breed a race of men on the average considerably superior —*by our present standards*—to any race of men now existing in respect of many quantities or attributes." Dr. Pearl does not mention nutrition in his method of control over the activities of human beings. But his book was written in 1922 when the knowledge of nutrition was nothing compared with what we know today.

Dr. Margaret Mead, the famous U.S. anthropologist in a talk before the World Federation for Mental Health in Berlin in 1956, expressed a need to give some thought to the mental health of world leaders who can decide disaster or prosperity for the world. She said that "wars begin in the minds of men," and that the mental health of individual statesmen is important for the maintenance of peace. But, not being a nutritionist, Margaret said nothing about nutrition as a factor in creating "safer" statesmen.

What Can You Expect From This Book?

You can expect a definite plan—a blueprint that you can follow, to be put into effect gradually. Chapter by chapter you will be given evidence about why some of the things you are doing are preventing you from using your brain as thoroughly as you otherwise might. Chapter by chapter you will be told what to do and what not to do in order to get the full potential out of your "gray matter." And if you do these things we feel that not only will there be a great improvement in your mental capacity and ability, but you will live longer . . . because great mental power, with few exceptions, is associated with good health. In other words the mind is part of the body—a healthy body, in the full sense, means a healthy mind. We might also say it is easier for a healthy person to do a certain number of hours of mental work, than for a person who is not that healthy. This book will enable you to work your mind longer, before mental fatigue sets in, and it will give you the power to think deeper!

For whom is this book written? . . . for presidents of nations, for kings, for Einsteins, for college professors, for hewers of wood and drawers of water, and for the people in every category and profession of life. Very few persons are exempt from gaining some results if they follow the method outlined in this book.

1

Eat Meat for Superior Mental and Physical Health

This chapter will show you the first step you must take in a program of building up your mental and physical ability. You must be sure that you eat some meat or fish every day—also eggs! Only in this way can you get the right quality of protein with which to stoke your mental fires properly! If you have been a vegetarian up to this point you must change over to meat-eating at once. The sooner you do this the quicker will you attain that dynamic quality in your thinking and doing which will make you a superior person.

MEAT PROTEIN is a most important building block in your program of attaining the highest possible mental power. Keep the starch and sugar content of your diet at a minimum. The reasons for this will be explained in the Chapter (2) on sugar. Eat as much meat and fish as you possibly can.

The distinguished English psychiatrist, Dr. Charles Mercier (who aroused Freud's anger by referring to his work as *Freudian fairy tales*) described mental cases that were caused by diets too high in starch and sugar, and too low in meat. He obtained sensational cures by changing the diets of these mentally unbalanced people, having them cut down on starch and sugar and eating more meat. Dr. Mercier found that inadequate meat in the diet leads to a confusion of the mind.

18

He referred to cases of people who ate little or no meat as saying, "I feel muddled and dazed," or "A wave of confusion comes over me," etc.

I recall my first visit with a well-known vegetarian, a prolific writer on health subjects. He seemed terribly sad and woebegone—almost on the verge of tears. He was wearing shoes made of cloth as he would not be a part in any way of the slaughter of animals. He wanted to join our staff. I did not hire him. Although he wrote high-sounding scientific articles on the vegetarian diet, he was much too verbose. He did not seem to me to be normal.

What About George Bernard Shaw?

Take the case of George Bernard Shaw—a vegetarian, but a very angry man. I feel that it was his lack of animal protein that made him so irritated with the world. He once said, "I want people to be sufficiently discontented to feel that there is something to live for." *His* was a philosophy of discontent, which I am almost sure stemmed from his unhappy diet. But because he did not eat meat, Shaw overly indulged himself in sugar and starch-containing pastry, candy, and bread. In Theatre Arts (October, 1960), Shaw is described as being at a party, chattering and eating caramels in some back drawing room.

In London many years ago I bought from an autograph dealer, and still have in my possession, a penned list of foods in the handwriting of Mrs. Shaw, which was given in advance to chefs at hotels where Shaw would stay. It listed the kind of foods he would eat. It specifically mentions "puddings, pastry, and dessert like other people," probably meaning ice-cream and such.

Shaw once said, "I like fighting successful people, attacking them, rousing them, trying their mettle, kicking down their castles. . . . One learns from it." There are more gentle and humane ways of teaching than kicking people in the teeth!

Had Shaw eaten thick beef-steaks every day his body chemistry might have been different. He might have been more contented and less vicious in his writings. He might then have been submerged in the competition of the writings of hundreds of other good authors and playwrights. It is conceded that Shaw had a great manner of writing, and that he was capable of magnificent prose, but so were thousands of other English masters of prose, who wrote and were forgotten.

Why Meat Is Superior

Meat's superiority over vegetables is due to the fact that its protein is a *complete* protein; it contains all the essential amino acids in good distribution. This is not true of any vegetables except soya beans. Our organs are made up mainly of protein and we need good protein to keep their tissues in good repair, as they are constantly breaking down and wearing out.

A second most important fact about meat's superiority is the quick and full digestibility. A dog will gulp down a piece of meat, but not any vegetables. Actually, in man as well as dog, meat does not have to be chewed. Full digestion of it occurs naturally in the stomach. Thus, all of its components are broken down thoroughly and are better absorbed. This does not happen with plant foods.

Vegetarianism's Effect on Sex

A serious disadvantage of vegetarianism is its effect on sex. It has a tendency to dampen the sexual desire, to subdue it. Evidence seems to show that a virile man's health goes hand in hand with a virile sexual capacity. There is also evidence which shows that senility in old age is accompanied by a significant reduction in sexual power. In healthy old age, there have been cases where men lived to be over 100 and still had potent sexual powers.

In Bernard Shaw's *Dear Liar,* Mrs. Patrick Campbell, one of Shaw's "flames," told him right out that it was only his vegetarianism that kept him from being a threat to female virtue.

In a review of Shaw's work in the New York Times (May 5, 1961) the writer said, "The trouble with Shaw was that his Cleopatra did not have much sex. Shaw's idea of Caesar was what Shaw would have done if he had found Cleopatra." He probably would have expounded about how much more satisfying a carrot was than a piece of mutton.

There can be no question that the lack of meat acts to subdue the carnal fires of sex. Possibly it is due to a deficiency of vitamin B, because meat is much more abundant in this vitamin than the general run of vegetables. Dr. Benjamin Sieve of Boston (Journal of the A.M.A. March 24, 1945) is quoted as saying that the B complex of vitamins are associated with the body's manufacture of sex hormones. You will also discover when you read Chapter (8) on vitamin B how important this vitamin is to the well-being of the nerves that spark the action of the brain. Incidentally, the diet outlined in this book is a specific for the maintaining of a healthy sexual set-up in the body.

Famous Men Tried It

Benjamin Franklin as a young man was a vegetarian for a short period from the humanitarian standpoint, although he didn't go so far as to wear cloth shoes. He was cured when on a fishing pier he saw a catch being slit open, and in the innards of the big fish he saw little fish.

Said Benjamin, "If the big fish can eat the little fish, then I can eat fish of any size."

. In my opinion, the man was rationalizing. He was fed up and was looking for a way out! Spencer, the essayist, tried vegetarianism for a year, and claimed he had to throw away practically everything he wrote during that period.

The fact that strict vegetarians are subjecting themselves to possible mental damage is brought out in *The British Medical Journal* (June 16, 1962). It deals with a form of vegetarianism called *veganism*, which excludes *all* animal matter, eggs, milk, butter, etc. It was found that, "Although most of the vegans were clinically normal, the electro-encephalographic evidence suggests that occult damage to the central nervous system is taking place, and that this form of diet may produce subtle cerebral changes that are not recognizable by ordinary clinical methods."

What saved Shaw from this fate is that he ate eggs!

In studying man you will find that the meat-eating races have always conquered the non-meat eaters. And it is the same in the animal world. The wolf and the fox keep the rabbit in subjection. The horse will not run out of a burning stable, but you won't catch a lion or tiger staying there under such conditions. The vegetarian will say, look at the gorilla! Yes, look at him—an extremely stupid creature albeit very strong physically.

As I have often said, vegetarians may be stronger, they may run faster and climb higher quicker, but they are left behind when it comes to the dynamic mental aggressiveness that is needed in business, science, government, general education, etc. If you have a "big" job, don't prejudice your position by going vegetarian. I can't see that young

General Electric Company president I mentioned in the preface holding down his job on a vegetarian basis.

Don't Forget Eggs

So rule number one in our system to get the full use out of our brain is to eat plenty of meat, as well as other high protein items like fish and eggs, the latter being considered an excellent form of protein. Don't worry about the cholesterol content of the egg, because egg yolk is also rich in lecithin, which is the antidote to cholesterol. It emulsifies it, or breaks it up into tiny particles which are absorbed into the blood, preventing it from accumulating on the walls of the blood-vessels. The word *lecithin* derives from the Greek *lekothos,* and means the yolk of an egg. Lecithin is found in the nerves of the brain and our diet should be rich in it.

The whole cholesterol controversy to me has not been viewed properly. To me what counts is not cholesterol, but the general fat content of the diet. In America, the diet contain 40 percent fat—in Italy, only about 20 percent. Italians suffer less than one-half the heart disease deaths that we do, so get the content of fat in your diet down by at least a half. But to do this don't cut out nature's number one protein, the egg. This is a wonderful food in its protected package, a seed of life with potent nutrition in it, waiting for the emergence of the little chick that must live off it for a few days. Cut out milk, cheese, ice-cream, and other such negative items of diet, and you can forget about the cholesterol bugaboo. But eat two eggs every day and you will help build your mental power!

Regarding animal protein—meat and fish that is—eat only the fresh kinds. Shun processed meats, delicatessen, smoked or canned meats, salami, pastrami, corned beef, hot dogs, etc. Most of this kind of meat is heavily treated with toxic chemical additives for various reasons. In Iceland, cancer of the digestive system was traced to the common habit of smoking fish, a result of limited refrigeration over the winter. Iceland has about the highest cancer rate in the world. But to see the evidence of why chemical additives are harmful to the mind see Chapter (13) called *Chemicals in Food.* These chemicals are vitamin destroyers in the body, thus weakening its resistance to disease, and preventing many organs from functioning properly. Their general effect is to destroy good health, and this, of course, has a harmful effect on the brain.

Regarding fish, we recommend only the deep sea kind, such as flounder, haddock, cod, mackerel, tuna, rose fish, etc. Fish from inland waters are tainted from man's pollutions, from his sewage, from the discharge of the chemical wastes of factories, and from the poisonous chemical fertilizers and pesticides that wash off the land into creeks and rivers.

2

It Pays to Shun Sugar

You must cut out the use of white and brown sugar, and any products that contain them. The overuse of such products, strange to say, can produce a condition of low blood sugar which lowers the brain's efficiency. Sometimes it leads to mental troubles. The elimination of the refined sugars will give you more physical and mental energy, and may do away with headaches. It will also reduce tooth cavities to the vanishing point.

Some sports authorities advise the taking of white sugar to give extra energy in sport contests. This has been proven to be a fallacy. It does give additional energy for the moment, but then sets up a craving for more and more sugar. In the end, it will destroy athletic ability.

IF YOU WISH to develop mentally, one of the worst foods you can eat is white sugar, and white sugar products. There must be no candy, no ice-cream, no soda pop, no cookies, cakes, and pastries generally. Item by item you must rout these foods out of your diet. In their place, substitute fruits and sweet vegetables like the sweet potato, carrots, beets, etc.

There is a peculiar fact in connection with white sugar consumption. In consuming a lot of such sugar, instead of raising the blood sugar, in many cases it reduces it, causing a very low blood sugar content which in many cases leads to mental confusion and break-downs.

In a letter a doctor wrote to the editor of *The British Medical Journal* (June 22, 1963), he asks if it would be advisable to check all admissions to mental hospitals for low sugar. The reply is, "It is important constantly to keep in mind the possibility of a psychiatric state being due to an organic condition such as hypoglycemia," meaning low blood sugar.

But how is it that an intake of too much sugar can cause a condition of low sugar in the blood? The answer is that in order to prevent too much sugar from suddenly flooding into the circulation, the pancreatic gland secretes insulin which neutralizes the sugar excess. Overindulgence in sweets—especially the quickly absorbable ones like candy, ice-cream, cakes, sodas, etc.—cause a frantic over-stimulation of the pancreas. It becomes overworked, and loses its ability to work with precision. It over-functions; that is, errs on the plus side. Too much insulin is made, not enough sugar remains, and the level of sugar in the blood falls sharply. There are millions upon millions of persons suffering from low blood sugar in the U.S. on account of the national jitterbug diet.

If you wish to read up on this subject, get *Body, Mind and Sugar*, by E. M. Abrahamson, M.D., and A. W. Pezet (Henry Holt, 1953). The list of diseases which Dr. Abrahamson finds related to low blood sugar is long—alcoholism, migraine headaches, stomach ulcers, allergies, hay fever, asthma, fatigue, eczema, rheumatic fever, neuroses, suicide tendencies, etc., the last two conditions coming under the subject of our book. Dr. Abrahamson has found that adjusting the low blood sugar does away with the symptoms.

Usually, sufferers from low blood sugar have been told they suffer from everything from coronary thrombosis to brain tumor, epilepsy, gall bladder disease, appendicitis, hysteria and every sort of neurosis; in many cases they have been told that their trouble is "all in the mind," which is more truth than poetry.

Dr. Abrahamson outlines some of the symptoms of low blood sugar—fatigue, dizziness, headaches, and hunger pangs. These are some of the immediate indications that cells in the brain and the nervous system are exhausted and crying for sugar—*glucose* sugar, that is, the sugar manufactured in the human body.

A Case of Low Blood Sugar

In his book, Dr. Abrahamson describes the case of P.J., a woman of 48 who had suffered from claustrophobia and loss of memory (among other things), for 15 years. She went through psychoanalysis, and although Dr. Abrahamson later found her suffering from low blood sugar, the psychiatrist gave her shock treatments and injections of insulin which lowered still further her blood sugar. She became worse and lost her desire to live. She tried two more psychiatrists with no results. Then she found Dr. Abrahamson, who discovered that she was suffering from low blood sugar. He placed her on a diet high in protein and low in refined starches and sugar. "Within a week she began to feel better, both physically and emotionally. In two weeks she was able to travel alone, which had been impossible for her for years." Today she is cured.

What about the fallacy that sugar is needed for energy? It creates a false energy that lasts only a few moments, then causes a desire for more energy to appease the fatigue created by the previous dose of sugar.

Mary Haworth in her column in *The N.Y. Journal American* had been lauding Dr. Abrahamson's book. Here is a letter published in her column on April 15, 1957:

Dear Mary Haworth:

   Two and a half years ago I read in your column about the book, *Body, Mind and Sugar* (Holt Publishers), by Dr. E. M. Abrahamson and A. W. Pezet.

   I promptly bought it and nearly cried from joy when I read the familiar symptoms of my miserable state of utter weakness—with a correct interpretation put on my illness, for the first time.

   Before I had finished reading the book I promised myself that if the corrective diet, described by the authors, would return me to normal health, I would write a letter of thanks to your column—and to the authors of the volume.

   It is this promise that I am fulfilling today. I thank you from the bottom of my heart for bringing this book to my attention. During miserable years I was an absolutely useless person; and doctors in five different countries couldn't help me. Then nothing short of a miracle happened, when the sugarless diet changed me completely—and I am now as full of zest and energy as I could wish.

   My thankfulness is eternal.

                                        Yours faithfully—D.N.

Here is another letter Miss Haworth published on the same date:

Dear Mary Haworth:

I would like to take this opportunity to congratulate you for the wonderful work you are doing—particularly, in calling attention to such a timely book as *Body, Mind & Sugar* (Holt), by Dr. E. M. Abrahamson and A. W. Pezet. The editors of a national magazine are interested in a story about my wife, who was a so-called mental patient for some months and had been regarded as a hopeless case, and then was healed by the diet outlined in *Body, Mind and Sugar,* that counteracts hyper-insulinism (blood sugar starvation).

Then follows comment by Mary Haworth herself:

"I haven't kept any file of testimonial mail on this subject, but four letters of endorsement stand out in my memory.

"The earliest came from the wife of a Naval officer, about four years ago. She was the first person to call my attention to Abrahamson and Pezet's book. The second was from a doctor's wife, who reported that her husband had been practicing, successfully, for some 20 years, along the lines of Dr. Abrahamson's findings—namely, that many symptoms labeled neurotic or even psychotic are linked to blood sugar imbalance.

"The third letter came from a doctor, who firmly lauded the book as a boon to his health; and the fourth, from a staff employee of a treatment center in the Middle West, who wrote that clinic members had become firm fans for the book—as an urgently needed supplement to their store of therapeutic knowledge."

Another Case of Low Blood Sugar

Another physician who has demonstrated a relationship between low blood sugar and mental disturbance is Sam E. Roberts, M.D., who in his book, *Ear, Nose, and Throat Dysfunctions* (Charles C. Thomas Co., Springfield, Ill.), devotes a whole chapter to low blood sugar. Dr. Roberts believes that many patients who go from doctor to doctor seeking cures for nervousness, anxiety, and exhaustion are suffering from low blood sugar. Instead of being told they are neurotics, they should be given a diet to overcome the low blood sugar condition. He says that rapid fluctuations in blood sugar common in this kind of condition often give rise to many bizarre symptoms that suggest mental disorders. "Before the final diagnosis of any nervous or mental disease is made, the patient should be given the therapeutic test for at least three months. As previously stated, I am certain that the population of our institutions for patients with nervous and mental disturbances would be greatly reduced if this regimen were followed."

Some of the patients that Dr. Roberts saw had been to their family doctor, who discovered the low blood sugar condition and described a diet high in sugar to correct it. But naturally this only worsened the condition.

May I offer the experience of a dentist, Dr. Donald Shriber of Los Angeles, who in the Sept. 1958 issue of *Modern Nutrition* tells about a patient, an 8-year-old boy named Tommy Smith. "He would return to my office every three months with from three to five new cavities to be filled. This continued over a long period of time, resulting in a filling in every tooth including the permanent ones. At first each appointment with him was the same—kicking, biting, and screaming. I could have rewarded that child with the Empire State Building and still would be bitten, kicked, and screamed at. In desperation, since I had to preserve my hands (which to me are very valuable), my glasses, ear drums, and nervous system. I prescribed a sugar-and-white-flour free diet for the boy, mostly for my own protection. It worked. Six months later there were no new cavities and only one cavity a year later. I was amazed at the child's behavior while on this program. Here was a happy contented child, who six months before had been a pint sized tornado. His mother revealed some more facts which were amazing to me at this time. The school authorities had been seriously considering placing the child in the 'retarded group' beacuse of his inability to keep up with the class. He also had continually quarreled with his sister; later there were only a few occasional spats. Before, he was having one cold after another and frequent sore throats; recently he had only one cold and no sore throats. His mother had had to continually watch his bowels; now they moved normally without laxatives. The correlation between tooth decay, the common cold, sore throats, constipation, and lack of interest in his school studies seemed important to me. It was quite obvious that the absence of sugar in this boy's diet apparently was the factor which was contributing to the solution of the above dilemma!"

The Case of Adolf Hitler

Adolf Hitler makes a startling case for the harmful effect of sugar on an individual, for Hitler was a "sugar drunkard." This, no doubt, is one of the factors that contributed to his becoming a restless, shouting, trigger-brained, raving maniac. It caused him to lose his sense of values. There can be no question that Hitler suffered from low blood sugar, due to an overconsumption of sugar.

Ernst Hanfstaengl, Hitler's personal pianist, wrote a book about him called *Unheard Witness* (Lippincott), which throws a great deal of light on Hitler's diet. He showed that Hitler could never get enough of his favorite whipped-cream cakes. There was always a box of candy near him. He could not drink wine unless he put sugar in it. In the early days of his career, when Hitler was in jail, his friends deluged him with boxes of candy, knowing of his predilection for them.

In *The Rise and Fall of the Third Reich* (Simon and Schuster), author William L. Shirer confirms the fact that Hitler craved sweets. Here are several excerpts from this book:

"On the afternoon of Sunday, January 29th, while Hitler was having coffee and *cakes* with Goebbels and other aides, Hermann Goering, President of the Reichstag and second to Hitler in the Nazi Party, burst in and informed them categorically that on the morrow Hitler would be named Chancellor." (p. 4.)

"At the swank Adlon Hotel, where the party was put up in the best suite, there were chocolates for Miss Hacha (daughter of the President of Czechoslovakia)—a personal gift of Adolf Hitler, who believed that everyone else shared his craving for sweets." (p. 444.)

There were several other references in this book illustrating Hitler's intense passion for sugar foods. In the book, *Hitler's Secret Conversations*, there is a discussion with Admiral Fricke in which Hitler said, "Not long ago I drank for the first time in my life a really good wine, with an extraordinary bouquet. The drinkers with me said it was too sweet."

The Nurse Who Killed Babies

How many of you remember the case of Virginia B.

Jaspers, a very obese nurse who killed three babies that were placed in her care? She shook them to death because they got on her nerves by refusing to take their formula. She broke the leg of a fourth infant and inflicted a head injury on a fifth. When an inquisitive newspaper reporter interviewed her, he said she showed a child's passion for ice-cream and soda pop. She was a sugar addict and had to have a box of candy at her side all the time. All day long she drank sweet carbonated beverages.

Another example of criminals who were slaves to sugar are the cases of the four women who were executed for murder in the State of California in the last 20 years or so. The most recent is Mrs. Elizabeth Duncan who killed her pregnant daughter-in-law. Here again a curious journalist, Eddy Jo Bernal, analyzed the character of these four women and found many similarities. These are his words in the *Los Angeles Herald Examiner* of August 12, 1962: "All liked desserts and sweets. . . . All the women liked candy and ice-cream. Mrs. Spinelli ate ice-cream and pie the night before she died. Mrs. Peete nibbled candy and offered a box of it to reporters and photographers the day before she was executed. Barbara Graham's last meal was a hot fudge sundae. Mrs. Duncan throughout her trial was munching on Life-savers and peppermints."

In *The British Medical Journal* (Jan. 18, 1958), there is described a case of a young man who murdered his mother. Upon examination he was found to be suffering from low blood sugar. There should be a sugar study follow-up in connection with the commission of all major crimes. In fact, the whole diet of every arrested criminal should be thoroughly checked.

A reader of *Prevention* magazine (of which I am the editor) writes: "Fiorello LaGuardia, one time mayor of New York City, used to eat Zabaglione for dessert almost every day. This is sherry wine, sugar, and egg yellow. Some of his closest long-time aides broke with him in his last term as mayor because he became so dictatorial."

In Zabaglione, sugar is the major ingredient.

In 1900, the average sugar consumption in this country was about 10 pounds per person. Today it is about 110 pounds per person, or eleven times as much, and it is still going up year by year, because the craving for it is like taking drugs. It may get so high one day, and low blood sugar may become so prevalent, that people will be shot down in the streets like dogs by sugar-crazed people. No one will be safe!

How to Do It!

So—go heavy on meat and fish and eat two eggs a day, but no white sugar at all, in any form whatever. This means no ice-cream, candy, cake, pastry, pies, no sugar in your coffee. Rice pudding is taboo because it is sugar treated. If made with honey it would be satisfactory.

Stewed prunes in the U.S. are acceptable. No sugar is used on them, but this is not so in Spanish-speaking countries. You can taste the difference.

For good sugar eat figs, apples, pears, sweet-potatoes, dates, etc. But even these should be consumed in moderation. In fruit the sugar is whole, and not refined as in white sugar. The white sugar is water-soluble and rushes right into the blood stream without being digested. The whole sugar of fruit contains vitamins and minerals.

It is known, for example, that sugar cane as a whole product is healthy. Natives who eat large quantities of it don't get dental caries. But when white sugar extracted from sugar cane is eaten it will cause caries. Bear in mind that too much of the whole sugar of fruit can be fattening.

It will be more difficult for some to give up sugar than it will for others. Therefore the problem must be carefully thought out and planned for. Do it gradually, perhaps. Cut it out item by item over a period of time. But as you begin to see benefits accruing, you will be encouraged to accelerate your pace. You will probably prove to your own satisfaction that white sugar does not furnish energy, as many people suppose; you will probably wind up with *more* energy. You will no doubt have to over-do the fruit at the beginning. Take fruit to work so you won't have to eat a sugar dessert at lunch.

You may have a little trouble for a few days, perhaps a week, but persevere, and soon you will be able to pass an inviting pastry window without getting excited! In a short time you will feel your body regenerating itself—and in time it will give you more mental energy.

3

Don't Use Salt—Key to Greater Brain Power

Eliminate added salt from your cuisine. There is sufficient natural salt in your food to take care of your body's needs. Salt, by waterlogging the blood vessels, reduces their ability to carry sufficient oxygen and other nutrients to the brain. Salt users are only standing in the way of enabling their brains to function efficiently. The fact that man needs extra salt in his food is an outmoded idea. It has been proven wrong both for man and animal.

IN THIS AND the next chapter we will discuss the use of salt and tobacco as factors that reduce mental efficiency, showing you what happens to the blood vessels feeding the brain when you use salt or indulge in smoking. Salt and tobacco cause a shrinkage in the space in the blood vessels through which the blood must flow.

Actually, the width of the blood vessels varies in different persons because of factors of birth and environment. Some persons have wider-than-average blood vessels, so that even if cholesterol does get on the vessel walls there is still room for the blood to circulate freely. These, no doubt, are the ones who can violate all the rules of health and still live to a ripe old age. Churchill, no doubt, must have had wide arteries to begin with. But the narrow-arteried people get struck down by the first ill-wind that blows.

Women on the average have wider blood vessels than

men, which may be one of the reasons why they live five to six years longer than men.

Dr. Samuel Rosen, of Columbia University's College of Physicians and Surgeons, let a medical expedition into the Sudan where he found a tribe with a wonderfully-developed sense of hearing, and commenting on it in *Newsweek* he said, "Narrowed arteries to the inner ear might dull hearing by impeding the blood flow to the cochlea—the shell-shaped organ within the skull which houses the auditory nerve endings." Evidently these Sudanese had wide arteries going to the cochlea.

Wide-Arteried People

A Virginia doctor claims that overweight is not necessarily a health hazard. He bases his theory on the fact that there are fat old people. But perhaps these fat old people have wide arteries? The narrow-arteried fat people have long since died off. So don't be a narrow-arteried fat person!

A most significant piece of research was done at the Rothschild Hadassah University Hospital in Jerusalem, and reported in *The Lancet* (June 29, 1957). It was found that where there were very thin capillaries in people, a large percentage of them had high blood pressure and severe heart disease.

Metchnikoff in his work discovered that girls with very narrow arteries were of a very sickly type—almost green-complexioned and affected with serious diseases.

In this book we are interested in the working of the mind, and what we can do to improve it. Therefore, we would like to know, first, do narrow blood vessels retard its operation in any way, and secondly, if so, what can we do about it?

Many pieces of research have been done in mental institutions to check on whether mentally disturbed patients have any differences in capillary width and shape from normal persons. I will discuss one of them done by Hildegard Rand Maricq, M.D., at the Veterans Administration Hospital, at Lyons, N.J. (*Circulation,* March '63). The experiment involved 92 schizophrenics and 60 normal persons. There were distortions in the finger-nail capillary patterns of all the mental patients, but none in that of the normal persons. Miss Maricq says of the schizophrenic group, "In most instances, the capillary blood flow appeared to be slower than normal. . . . Another striking feature repeatedly encountered was the presence of capillaries with no active circulation." Incidentally, it is a fact that if there is a condition of the capillaries in the nail bed it usually reflects a similar condition in the rest of the body.

Now what does this mean? It means that something a person has been doing has twisted the capillaries out of shape, so that the blood cannot circulate freely. It means also that we must examine our habits and be sure that we are not doing any of these things. It means further that we must seek ways to enlarge our blood vessels if they are narrow to begin with.

One way to do this is by exercise, which not only has the effect of dilating the blood vessels, but can actually create *new* capillaries. Exercise also oxygenates the blood vessels, and that is the end result we are wishing for—to feed oxygen and other nutrients to our various organs, glands and tissues, including the brain area.

What Salt Does to the Veins

The effect of using salt is to seriously reduce the inner area of all the blood vessels throughout the body. Salt is a pure chemical—sodium chloride—a highly soluble and very active compound which rushes into the water solution of the body without going through the process of digestion.

The fallacy exists that man must have extra salt in his diet in order to be healthy. Yet there are hundreds of millions of people all over the world who have never used salt, and still are perfectly healthy. Man does need *some* salt, but he can obtain it from the salt which is a natural component of most foods. The only reason animals will travel long distances to get salt is that they have learned to like the taste of it, just as is the case with people. It is not necessarily an intrinsic need of the animals. Members of the deer family in Maine never have had salt, and are as healthy as those in Montana which devour it in salt licks, and are always seeking more.

The use of salt prevents the full oxidation of the circulation passageways in the brain. I came across an article in *Connecticut Medicine* (Jan. '62) by Louis H. Nachum, M.D., which, while it deals with high blood pressure, talks about salt and its effect on the blood vessels. Dr. Nachum says that high blood pressure is due to an increase in the resistance to the flow of blood from the arteries into the capillaries, which are almost hair-like in measurement. Such increase is due to the narrowing of the artery passageways. Something happens, caused by something a person does, that narrows down the diameter of the arteries. Naturally, if blood has to push through a smaller space it must push harder against the resistance and against the walls of the arteries; that is what raises the pressure of the blood.

Sometimes the passageways of the small arteries become narrowed due to a nervous condition. Sometimes it is due to certain hormones secreted by some of the glands of the body. But it has also been proven that salt is a prominent cause of narrowing the artery passageways, and the consequent high blood pressure. That is why people with high blood pressure (or hyper-tension—which means too much tension) are told by doctors that they must eliminate table salt from their diet!

Dr. Nachum maintains that if salt is the cause of a certain kind of hyper-tension, then by restricting the use of salt there will result an increase in the diameter of the arteries, thus reducing the hyper-tension. According to Dr. Nachum, salt, because it encourages water-logging, causes a swelling of the walls of the blood-vessels, and a reduction in the size of the remaining space in the blood vessels, thus offering more pressure against the passage of blood, increasing the blood pressure.

I have presented this information to show that the use of table salt could impede the circulation of the blood in the brain and prevent sufficient oxygen from circulating there, which could lead to some kind of mental trouble.

Salt and Baldness

Now I would like to discuss another piece of medical research which implicates salt as a cause of a certain condition in the head, namely baldness. The doctor who did this work, Eugene Foldes, reported it in *ACTA*—Dermato —Venereologica, Vol. 35, p. 334, 1955. Dr. Foldes knew that an excess of certain elements, especially sodium, may accumulate in some tissues and interfere with the proper functioning of those tissues. He reasoned that an accumulation of sodium (salt is sodium chloride) in the scalp might disturb the function of those tissues in the growing of hair, and that this function might be improved by reducing the amount of sodium in these tissues.

Dr. Foldes did his experimental work with people by counting the number of hairs that fell out of their scalp every day. But in the case of his first experiment, a woman

62 years of age who complained of loss of hair, instead of having her eliminate salt from her diet, he gave her a *diuretic,* which is a drug that helps the body expel fluids through the urine, and this always carries a certain amount of salt out with it. In the first three weeks of the experiment this woman reduced her average daily hair loss by about 46 percent.

In the case of a male patient who had noticed an excessive loss of hair during the last three years, the treatment cut down hair loss by about 60 percent. Incidentally, in this experimental work, Dr. Foldes found that shampooing the hair is accompanied by a larger than average hair loss. Dr. Foldes discovered that adherence to a low salt diet significantly reduced the loss of hair, while after two days or more of unrestricted salt intake, the rate of loss of hair was always significantly increased.

Now if we relate Dr. Foldes' work with that of Dr. Nachum, we will come up with something. According to Dr. Nachum, salt reduces the size of the blood vessels in the body, including the head and brain. Thus, due to an impaired blood circulation in the scalp, there might result a failure to nourish the root hairs properly, and hair weakened in this way might fall out—this along with the effect of the accumulation of sodium, which interferes with the proper functioning of the tissues.

Size of Veins and Mental Disease

In cerebral arteriosclerosis, which is a thickening of the walls of the blood vessels in the brain causing intellectual deterioration and mental aberrations, we see another confirmation of the fact that reducing the size of the blood vessel passageways in the brain can affect the mind.

In *Highlights of Mental Health Research 1955,* issued by the Social Legislation Information Service, Inc., Washington, D.C., a study on mental health research by The National Institute of Mental Health is discussed. It states, "The research of a number of the Institute scientists is concerned with fundamental studies of the brain's blood circulation as another means of obtaining new knowledge of the brain's structure and function in health and disease. Disturbances in cerebral circulation are known to be among the basic causes of a number of neurological disorders, and may be at the root of mental diseases such as the senile psychoses. . . . Following adolescence, there is a more gradual but progressive reduction of the circulation throughout the remaining life span. What the reasons are for this decline are not yet known."

Dr. Masor, of whom we will speak later, has found that using salt can cause an enlargement of the thyroid, causing an interference with the transport of oxygen, which is why many under-active thyroid cases become mentally disturbed.

Let's not overlook the fact also that the chloride portion of salt can destroy vitamin E in the body, and, as will be shown later, this vitamin is of terrific importance to the well-being of the brain. For one thing, it helps to oxygenate the body and brain.

The use of salt is just a habit, and like any other habit, it can be eradicated with a little effort. Granted, you will miss it for a short time—perhaps for a week or so—but if you will try to avoid its use for a little while you will soon begin to wonder how you ever liked it!

IN REVIEW

Go strong on meat, fish, and eggs.
Eat as little as possible of carbohydrates.
No sugar.
No salt.

4

Smoking Reduces Thinking Ability

> *Tobacco and optimum brain power do not go together. If it means anything to you to get the utmost out of your mental set-up, throw away your cigarette, cigar, or pipe. They will all dull the keenness of your mind. Along with salt, tobacco constricts the blood vessels and destroys vitamin C. It slowly weakens every organ in the body, leading to cancer of the lungs and reducing the ability of the mind to act brilliantly. A good thinker is not a smoker, in spite of the outward appearance of the smoking man.*

WHILE ON THE subject of the blood vessels, and the importance of keeping them dilated, let us take a look at tobacco! Smoking definitely constricts the blood vessels! The famous Alton Ochsner, M.D. and President of the International Society of Surgery, once said that every time a cigarette is smoked, it is like putting a clamp on the blood vessels. It has been shown that smoking even one cigarette will constrict the arteries, veins, and capillaries, and to that extent will slow down the blood circulation in all parts of the body, including the brain.

A friend of mine, a heart case and a heavy smoker, was told to lay off smoking. He did, on and off. When he had a fatal heart attack, they found the stubs of cigarettes in his bathroom.

How does tobacco cause a contraction of the blood vessels? The theory is that nicotine over-stimulates the pituitary gland in the head, releasing a hormone which acts on the blood vessel walls. Smoking of only one or two cigarettes causes a release of from 3 to 190 milli-units of the hormone into the bloodstream. This work done by Dr. J. H. Burn of Oxford, who said that smoking definitely involves a degree of restriction of the coronary circulation. Also the head, Dr. Burns!

King George VI died because of a narrowed coronary artery that was not helped by cigarette smoking. His condition was aggravated by having to stand stiffly at public ceremonies. The king had to give up public appearances in 1948 because of the pain in his right leg caused by a narrowing of the arteries. He was suffering from Buerger's disease, which affects only heavy cigarette smokers. One night the blood slowed down in a narrowed coronary artery; because of this slowness, the blood thickened and a clot formed that killed him. His arteries were probably narrow to start with, and his smoking narrowed them still more. He should never have smoked.

Tobacco and Insanity

I would like to quote something written by a physician in 1892. L. Bremer, an M.D. stationed at the St. Vincent's Institution for the Insane of St. Louis, Missouri, read a paper before a medical society in which he said that the eminent German philosopher, Kant, "is said to have written in such an obscure and unintelligible style because he smoked and used snuff to excess. . . . It may look like overstating and exaggerating things, but I know whereof I speak when I say that tobacco, when habitually used by the young, leads to a species of imbecility which makes the juvenile smoker lie, cheat, and steal. . . . This kind of insanity I have observed in quite a number of cases at the St. Vincent's."

Talking about one of the boys at this institution, he goes on: "The father of one of them who looked upon his son only as an aggravated case of bad boy, told me that he himself had been smoking ever since his 10th year and that it never affected him. In reality, being only 45 years old, he was a wreck, physically and mentally, though he came of healthy stock. . . .

"Is it to be wondered at, that a drug (nicotine) which has such potent and palpable effects as to produce loss of coordination and unspeakable malaise, and, after the organism has become used to it, is capable of setting up well-known heart disturbances, amblyopia (dimness of vision), and even amaurosis (blindness), which in short possesses the characteristic qualities of a powerful nerve poison—is it a wonder if such drug, in spite of the warnings on the part of various organs, excessively and persistently used, finally produces one or the other form of insanity? A drug that can, as has been demonstrated, cause organic change in the optic nerve, which, I hardly need mention, is in reality not a nerve, but a protrusion or elongation of the brain itself, must certainly be capable of injuriously influencing other and functionally higher parts of the organ of the mind."

A More Modern Example

Now if Dr. Bremer is too old-fashioned for your blood I will give you something right up to the minute—1960 shall we say? An Associated Press dispatch of December 26, 1960 describes the work of a University of Maryland psychologist who studied the effect of cigarette smoking on the academic work of colleges students. This was done by Dr. Donald K. Pumroy, and it proved that the more a student smoked the lower was the quality of his school work.

The study was done with 204 freshmen. It was found that 119 non-smokers had an average grade of 1.98. Those who smoked half a pack of cigarettes a day averaged 1.92, those who smoked from half a pack to a full pack a day earned a grade of 1.61, while those who smoked more than a pack a day averaged only 1.38.

Let us look at the government's report, *Smoking and Health*. On page 370: "Salber reports that among boys from the Newton, Mass., public schools, non-smokers in every grade have a higher mean IQ than discontinued smokers, who have higher mean IQ's than smokers. . . . In the same study a high relationship was found between achievement scores obtained from school grades and non-smoking. . . . Earp found that more smokers than non-smokers among Antioch College students failed to graduate. . . ."

Let us look further into the government's report on smoking; page 366: "Non-smokers were found by one investigator to show greater social participation in organizations and to hold more offices—activities more associated with extro- than with introversion. . . . Most studies support the contention that neuroticism is associated with the smoking habit. . . . In a study by Matarazzo and Saslow, smokers report more psychosomatic symptoms than non-smokers. . . . In the English study by Eysenck, heavy, medium, and ex-smokers of cigarettes were found to have the largest number of psychosomatic disorders, non-smokers, the least."

Smoking Reduces Thinking Ability

So, there is some evidence that smoking depresses the mental abilities. Can this be the reason why so many students fear to go in for difficult subjects and the country is faced with a serious shortage of scientists, engineers, physicians, etc.? How many of these truants are pack-a-day smokers? How many smokers in industry are accepting full salaries and exerting only half of their mental potential?

Many persons who smoke don't seem to fear cancer of the lungs; that is too far away; but if they knew that it was making them only half a person in their mental relations with their fellow man *right now*, would they be deterred?

The use of salt and tobacco are contributory factors in the causation of nervous breakdowns. Salt, because it narrows the arteries and does not permit an adequate flow of blood to the brain region, preventing its full oxygenation. Therefore, the moment a person gets a nervous breakdown, the use of salt and tobacco should be stopped. Yet in mental hospitals the foods are usually seasoned with salt, and no attempt is made to prohibit smoking. I was amazed recently, in visiting a friend in a mental ward of a hospital, to see all of the patients smoking. In fact, they were chain smoking, lighting up one cigarette from another, because they were not allowed to have matches. Cigarettes they were permitted, but not matches!

Here is an interesting fact; the width of the blood vessels varies widely in different persons. Now, suppose a person has very narrow blood vessels to begin with, and he or she smokes and uses salt—is it not sheer insanity? These persons are not receiving proper medical guidance.

Chiropractic Treatments

One more thing: Since the circulation of blood in the head is so important, I suggest regular chiropractic treatments. This can greatly improve the blood circulation in the head region. The writer takes a chiropractic treatment once a week—but of course I am 66. For younger persons, whether they need it or not, a treatment once a month will never be regretted.

Another suggestion: try to sleep without a pillow. Bending the neck in sleep prevents the free flow of blood to the head.

In closing, may I also say that smoking destroys the vitamin C in the body. Every puff kills some vitamin C. Heavy smokers are terribly vitamin C deficient, and a vitamin C deficiency is one of the causes leading to mental disturbances, as will be described in the chapter on vitamin C.

IN REVIEW

Meat, fish, eggs—
Low on carbohydrates—
No sugar and salt—
No smoking—

5

The Myth That Alcohol
Reduces Tensions

Alcohol, salt, and tobacco are the three unwanted handmaidens, as far as a healthy intellect is concerned. Keep your drinking down to a bare minimum. I don't recommend teetotalism, but a drink once in awhile on a social occasion, provided there are not too many social occasions. The drunkard, could never be an intellectual genius. Cut down on your drinking at once if you are a drinker, and gradually get it down to as near to nothing as possible. Alcohol confuses the mind by destroying valuable vitamins that are needed to feed it.

MANY PERSONS entertain the idea that alcohol is something that can relax them, that it is the perfect antidote to the so-called mental tensions of our times, and thus will help to stave off a mental breakdown. Well, if you are susceptible to such thinking, I have news for you: this philosophy is not based on scientific fact. And I can prove it with scientific work that has been done in medical institutions.

Alcohol tends to reduce the blood flow and prevent the delivery of sufficient oxygen to the brain. Work was done in Finland by the State Alcohol Monopoly Research Laboratories, as reported in *The Quarterly Journal of Studies on Alcohol* (Dec. 1955), which showed that moderate or immoderate drinking of any kind of alcoholic beverages causes the red blood cells to stick to each other in clumps, which slows down the speed of the blood flow, thus reducing the oxygen supply to all the tissues of the body. All three, namely salt, tobacco, and alcohol, should be taboo to anyone who wishes to have a good oxygen supply available to the brain tissues at all times.

A Popular Fallacy

Many physicians believe that alcohol opens up the blood vessels, and is therefore good for heart patients. But the findings from three U.S. Public Health studies, published in the May 27, 1950 issue of the *Journal of the American Medical Association,* show differently. The authors found from electrocardiograms that alcohol does not open up the coronary (heart) arteries at all. They say that the prevailing idea that alcohol is good medicine for heart cases "should be drastically amended."

One of the researchers (Dr. Henry I. Russek) says that it might actually be dangerous, even though an ounce or so of whiskey often stops pain. There is danger that the alcohol will remove the warning signal which pain is supposed to give. Dr. Russek says, "The view that a glass of whiskey is the equivalent of a glyceryl trinitrate tablet for the patient with coronary disease should be rejected."

Says *Science News Letter,* June 3, 1950, commenting on this research:

> The whiskey, they found, did not prevent the changes in the electrocardiograms brought on by the exercise test, but the glyceryl trinitrate either completely prevented or significantly modified these changes.
>
> The whiskey did prevent the pain and other sensations of angina, however.
>
> Alcohol's effect in angina, they conclude, is due to its rapid action as a sedative. The tests with morphine bore this out. And while the sedative effect may be good for the patient having an attack of angina, it could be dangerous for a person to take whiskey before undertaking vigorous physical effort.
>
> The alcohol would not dilate his arteries, and would banish the danger signal of pain, thus perhaps putting him in the spot of undertaking more than his heart can stand. Sudden death or fatal seizure might be the result.

Alcohol Bad for the Red Corpuscles

In connection with alcohol causing the red corpuscles to clump together, the studies claim that this occurs even in the case of moderate drinking.

My oldest brother, Archie, who died of a heart attack at age 51, was one of those who took a little nip here and there actually because of his heart condition, by advice of his doctor, who believed that a little drinking would keep him alive. But he did it once too often. After supper one night, instead of resting, he decided to fix a chair. He had been artificially invigorated by a little nip and was falsely lulled into a state of security. He never finished the job. He keeled over in a fatal heart attack.

It was the same with my brother, Joe, another moderate drinker who did it "for his heart." A heart attack killed him at 56. I have seen many friends, who drank moderately on the advice of their physicians, die long before their allotted time. No sir! This moderate protective drinking is a dangerous fallacy!

Drinking and its effect on the heart is an important subject, but in this book we are concerned with its effect on the brain—and it *does* affect it. Quoting from *The American Practitioner and Digest of Treatment* (July, 1956): "This short study seems to indicate that psychotic reactions described as a result of cerebral arteriosclerosis may be precipitated by the toxic effect of alcohol, by malnutrition, etc."

Dr. Henry Brill, head of Pilgrim State Hospital (New York City), says one of the major causes of mental illness is chronic alcoholism with its accompanying lack of vitamins. The alcoholic does not eat proper food.

Alcohol Destroys Vitamin B

Here is an item from *Medical Press* (245/2:30-34) quoted in World Wide Abstracts (May, 1961): "Chronic alcoholics mostly suffer from severe malnutrition. The treatment of alcoholism involves a high protein and vitamin intake." It is not generally known, however, that every drink of an alcoholic beverage destroys some vitamin B in the body. The craving for alcohol, no doubt, starts with a vitamin B deficiency caused by an unbalanced diet. The first thing that is done with severe alcoholic cases when hospitalized is to give them massive doses of this vitamin. Alcoholism causes retrogression in mentality because a lack of vitamin B affects the nerves. When you drink at a party and get a little "high," you are temporarily insane.

It has been proven, also, that it is not the alcohol that causes the red nose—that is one of the symptoms of a vitamin B deficiency, caused by over-drinking.

The poet Thomas Ravenscroft wrote:

> Nose, nose, nose, nose
> And who gave thee that jolly red nose,
> Cinnamon, and ginger, nutmeg and cloves
> And that gave me my jolly red nose.

No, master Ravenscroft—it is not the cinnamon and ginger, or nutmeg and cloves, that give the jolly red nose. It is a vitamin B deficiency.

In a later chapter, there will be a discussion on vitamin B, and its effect on the mind.

Professor Roger R. Williams of the University of Texas, at a meeting of the American Chemical Society of Austin, Texas, on December 9, 1951, said that both alcoholism and mental disease stem from a dietary deficiency. Some people are born with dietary needs that are hard to satisfy, said Professor Williams. "As soon as they begin violating the rules of good nutrition by drinking quantities of alcoholic liquids, deficiencies develop. . . . People who get everything they need nutritionally never become alcoholics." He showed that laboratory animals on the best diets nutritionally do not drink alcohol. Those on deficient diets always do. Many human beings, said Professor Williams, have had their craving for alcohol completely abolished by getting their nutritional needs satisfied so that they need not drink in an uncontrolled manner any longer.

It seems that bars should give their customers vitamin B tablets instead of salted pretzels for free lunch.

Alcohol Damages the Liver

Excessive alcohol consumption can cause cirrhosis of the liver, and there is evidence that this is a major contributory cause in cases of mental disturbance. This was shown at the Jersey City Medical Center, by Dr. Carroll M. Leevy. He said that a poorly functioning liver frequently was associated with metabolism damage that in turn led to cerebral disturbances. In cirrhosis of the liver, ammonia and other noxious substances accumulate in the blood stream and bring about damage in the cerebral area by a sort of washing of the brain cells.

Another indictment which applies both to alcohol and tobacco is that they both help to lower the blood sugar level, which is a contributory factor to mental disease. Dr. Roberts, whose observations on low blood sugar were given in Chapter 2, has observed that many of his low sugar patients were chain smokers. So, for optimum mental and physical efficiency, be *practically* a teetotaler.

REVIEW

Eat meat, fish, eggs.
Be moderate on carbohydrates.
No sugar and salt.
No smoking, and no drinking.

6

How Vitamins Can Help You Get More Out of Life

If you are not a vitamin taker, make up your mind right now that your life is about to undergo a drastic change. You are going to become a vitamin taker. When you read the evidence in the next few chapters, you are bound to be convinced that many vitamins are specific as "brain foods," so to speak. The trouble is that man seems to be too busy to stop and take inventory as to what our commercial system of producing is doing to our food, how they have eliminated from it many valuable nutrients that the body sorely needs to operate both physically and mentally.

If you do not remedy this gap, not only will you not be able to attain maximum mental and physical power, but you are a sitting duck for any disease germ that wishes to attack you! You can kill two birds with one stone—good nutrition, including the taking of minerals.

THE BASIS of the Rodale system for keener mental ability and better health is an improvement in one's diet, and a prominent part in this system is the taking of extra vitamins. In spite of a mass of evidence that there is an insufficiency of vitamins in our diets, the medical profession generally does not favor the taking of vitamins. A certain doctor I read about advised a patient to get his vitamins with his knife and fork. How dangerous this advice is in these days of factory refinement of food, when the mass American diet reflects a lack of any semblance of nutritional intelligence, and when doctors themselves are dying so young. Generally speaking, it is quite impossible for the average person to get enough vitamins and minerals from his diet for many reasons. First we have the controversial matter of the organic versus the chemical fertilizer method of raising our food. There is evidence that the lower the soil fertility, the poorer the nutritional quality of our food. This is shown by the fact that in the Middle West, in a recent 10 year period, the protein content of the grains were down by 11 percent. It is shown in the experience with sugar beets in Utah, where chemical fertilizer practices have reduced the sugar content of the beets to such an extent that it has become uneconomic for many farmers to raise sugar beets. It is shown in the State of Delaware, where it has become almost impossible to raise tomatoes, because of the disease in them due to soil that lacks full fertility elements. The use of nitrogenous fertilizers is causing copper deficiencies, and the overuse of potash fertilizers is creating magnesium deficiencies. These minerals are badly needed in our nutrition and we must correct their deficiency by taking mineral supplements, for our knives and forks will be quite ineffective to accomplish this. A serious situation has recently developed in regard to cattle feed. Due to the overuse of chemical fertilizer nitrogen, it has been found that cattle are not able to absorb much vitamin A from the feed. The same holds true for people. A great vitamin A deficiency is developing in the public due to the greater artificialization of the method of growing our food. The public is consuming food products of marginal quality, and if they do not get *extra* vitamins and minerals, they are bound to become weakened both physically and mentally.

Over-Refinement of Food

It is also a fact that the over-refinement of food makes it lose much of its nutritive value. This includes the removal of the living germ from the wheat in making bread, and the consumption of white polished rice. The whole brown rice contains about 300 to 400 percent more of the B vitamins than the polished variety. Eggs for the market are produced without benefit of roosters and are infertile, lacking important hormones and other living elements. Instead of sugar being consumed in the wholeness of raw sugar cane, it is refined into a chemical compound with all its vitamins removed.

We consume only part of the animal, neglecting the vitamin-rich organs such as the brain, heart, liver, kidney, etc. Primitive people have learned to consume wholeness. We fragmentize our diet, and the parts we throw away are underlying causes of our serious nutritional deficiencies.

It is a known fact that "only one person in a thousand escapes malnutrition." (Howard Blakeslee, Wide World science editor, in the *N.Y. Times.*) This was the conclusion of a six-year survey published by the Ellen H. Richards Institute at Penn State University. All this stems from the ignorance of the public of the most elementary facts of nutrition, and of the necessity of protecting itself by taking vitamins.

Back in 1947 we bought greater quantities of foods that required peeling, washing, trimming, and home cooking. Now we leave the store with packages of instant mashed potatoes, dehydrated soups, and frozen TV dinners. These items of food weigh less per calorie supplied. The most important effect of these convenience foods is on our food preparation habits. Women no longer want to take the time necessary to prepare fresh foods in the home. The number of hours that the average woman spends in preparing meals has dropped greatly in the past 15 years. What effect has this trend had on our intake of vitamins?

Green Vegetables

There also seems to be a drop in the consumption of leafy green vegetables. Our consumption in this category for the years 1947-49 was 98 pounds, and by 1960 it had dropped all the way to 80 pounds. When you realize that the average portion of spinach, for example, contains 10,680 units of vitamin A, you can see how a decline of almost 20 percent in our consumption of green and yellow vegetables can have a drastic effect on the amount of vitamin A we get.

Cabbage consumption has gone from 10.4 pounds per person in 1956 to 9.4 pounds in 1960. In the same period, carrots went from 6.8 pounds down to 5.3 pounds. While we used 16.5 pounds of lettuce and escarole in 1956, the amount dropped to 15 pounds in 1960. The fact that even the salad craze has not been able to stem the decline in the use of lettuce, carrots, and cabbage, is significant indeed.

Celery is down from 7.3 pounds per capita in 1956 to 6.7 pounds in 1960. Sweet potatoes—extremely rich in vitamin A—have taken an alarming drop in favor, from 7.6 pounds in 1956 to 6.2 pounds in 1960. Dry edible beans and peas have gone from 8.7 pounds in 1956 to 7.8 pounds in 1960. And bear in mind that I am not comparing one good year with one bad year. In almost every case there has been a steady and distinct decline in the consumption of these foods.

It is not surprising, therefore, that a nation-wide study made by the Household Economics Research Division of the Department of Agriculture, in 1955, showed that "nearly half of the nation's families used food that provided less than current allowances of the National Research Council in one or more nutrients."

Destruction in the Kitchen

We need extra vitamins and minerals because of the way we destroy vitamins and minerals in our kitchens. Let's take the case of what we do to the carrot before we eat it. The first thing we do is to throw away the top greens. This part has far greater nutritional value than the pulpy lower part. It contains vitamin K, for example. Before it came to us it was stored for some time, which causes it to lose vitamins. The housewife scrapes off the skin, wherein resides a large portion of the minerals. In many cases the carrots are soaked for a long time, causing some loss of the natural sugar, all the B vitamins, vitamin C and P, and much of the minerals except calcium.

If the carrots are shredded there is a loss of 20 percent of the vitamin C, and an additional 20 percent if used on a salad and allowed to stand for an hour before eating. This loss is due to oxidation; that is, the air penetrating the carrot.

Cooking destroys vitamins, and if salt is placed in the water, there is a greater loss in vitamin C. If carrots are frozen and thawed slowly, vitamin C is lost. So how much of the vitamin and mineral content of the carrot is preserved for one of those who gets his vitamins with his knife and fork?

And so it goes not only with the carrot but with many other items in our diet. Toast, for example, starts with the devitalized white flour; this is baked, and much of its remaining vitamins are destroyed. But when this baked bread is again subjected to heat in toasting, the last vestige of nutrition is all but eliminated. We make casseroles in which food is cooked two or three times. We recook leftovers that have hung around for weeks in the refrigerator —losing vitamins every day. In some foods, a single cooking destroys more than 50 percent of the vitamins. We should eat more *raw* food, but we don't.

The average person rarely eats raw foods. He even prefers his nuts roasted. His attitude on eating raw peas is that it is something done by food faddists. The same applies to carrots and turnips. Such so-called normal people should protect themselves by taking vitamins and minerals.

Destruction in the Factories

If food were handled naturally and not tampered with so much in the factories, it would be a different matter. In the factories food is bleached, colored, dehydrated, hydrolized, homogenized, emulsified, pasteurized, gassed, preserved chemically, and canned. Not only is there danger from the toxic qualities of these processes, but such toxicities are known to be destructive of vitamins, which are fragile substances that easily combine with other substances to form emasculated compounds. We also take in many elements harmful to vitamins in our drinking water —chlorine, aluminum, sulphates, carbon, hydrated lime, fluoride, and several others which the water-works manager is permitted to use in an emergency.

An additional important reason why we must take vitamins is the nature of the sedentary life we lead. Primitive man didn't need extra vitamins because he ate a lot of raw, fresh, wild, unprocessed food that was full of vitamins. Also, he was on the move most of the time. From morning to night he was out of doors, moving, working, and sweating, which gave him such a well-working digestive apparatus that it enabled him to absorb the maximum of vitamins from his food.

But modern man, with his ulcers, colitis, and other intestinal diseases, and his imperfect digestion, does not get the maximum out of his food. Sir Robert McCarrison, a great English nutrition researcher, has spoken of the "colonic lamentations of our civilization." He was comparing us with Hunzas of India, among whom he lived for 10 years. They are a primitive type of civilization, working all day and eating simple unprocessed food. They need no vitamin supplements. They are one of the healthiest peoples on earth.

We must not overlook the fact that some of the vitamin B is made by bacteria in the intestine, but a reduced amount will be manufactured in an intestine weakened by the way of living of a modern sedentary person. This reduces the amount of the intestinal flora. Such a person must take extra vitamin B or he will not be able to face up to the rigors of our way of life. Vitamin B is required for the health of the nerves. These vitamin B-deficient people are perhaps the ones who are always ranting against the stresses and strains of our times. If a person is well-nourished, he can withstand these stresses and strains without breaking down.

Vitamin Antagonists

We must take vitamins to restore those we destroy by our daily practices. Smoking destroys vitamin C, and drinking alcoholic beverages uses up some of the body's vitamin B. Coffee also drains some of the B vitamins out of our body. A diet overcharged with artificial sweets cuts in on the B vitamins. Chlorine in our drinking water destroys vitamin E in the body. Bridges' *Dietetics for the Clinician* says so on page 91. Chlorine dioxide used in bread has the same result. Vitamin E is also destroyed by rancid oil or fat in the diet. Inorganic iron compounds likewise destroy vitamin E. This is the kind of iron given in cases of anemia. Sterility, muscular dystrophy, and coronary disease may result from vitamin E deficiencies.

Raw fish is a robber of thiamin, one of the B vitamins. So if you eat raw clams and oysters, your body is being depleted if a goodly store of its thiamin. It is interesting to note that the Japanese, who are great eaters of raw fish and polished rice, have a rather low life expectancy.

Various kinds of chemicals are known to destroy vitamins. A widely used chemical sterilizer, ethyleneoxide, used extensively in the food industry, destroy the B vitamins, even though all the chemical is removed after treatment.

Chemically fertilized potatoes have a tendency to turn black, so the restaurants have to use anti-darkening chemicals like sodium bisulphite which destroys the vitamin B (thiamin). The loss is anywhere from 11 to 47 percent according to test.

In a recent study in South Carolina (*Charleston Evening Post*, December 1, 1960), it was found that almost half the meat products in the State "contained an injurious

addition commonly called *dynamite*." This is sodium
sulphite, which is the basic ingredient of washing and
cleansing detergents. The Commissioner of Agriculture
of the State, Wm. L. Harrelson, said, "Pure Food and
Drug officials claim that continuous consumption of
sodium sulphite destroys some of the body vitamins essential to the good health of human beings." This chemical
is found mostly in ground meat such as hamburgers, pork
sausages, chili meat, and cooked beef rounds.

Drugs Destroy Vitamins

Drugs are great brigands in robbing the body of vitamins. Estrogen, a hormone administered in certain diseases, cuts down three of the body's B vitamins—thiamin,
riboflavin, and niacin.

The barbiturates (sleeping pills) block the progress of
carbohydrate metabolism, and so add to the difficulty of
the body's absorption of thiamin.

Medicines given for malaria destroy vitamin B_2, or
riboflavin. The sulfa drugs upset the process of manufacturing B vitamins in the intestines. This is why pneumonia
patients, who get large doses of sulfa drugs, are left in a
state of terrible depression because of vitamin B depletion,
and this can go on for years unless corrected.

Penicillin and chloromycetin destroy niacin, and some
people are taking penicillin all the time. Arsenic and sulfa
compounds destroy P-amino-benzoic acid, a B vitamin.
Arsenic residues occur widely on fruits and vegetables—
residues of insecticides.

Mineral oil, used as a laxative, destroys vitamins A, D,
E, and K. Fluorides destroy the enzyme phosphatase,
upon which many vital processes in the body depend,
including its handling of vitamins.

A long list of other vitamin-destroying drugs could be
given, but it would make this book too technical if we
included them all. Suffice it to say that Americans by the
millions are using these drugs regularly, and so there is a
profound need to restore the vitamins which they remove
from their bodies.

Chemicals Destroy Vitamins

There are many chemicals all about us in our daily
environment which destroy or inactivate vitamins. Carbon
monoxide from car exhausts, sulphur compounds from
chimney smoke, tobacco smoke, and miscellaneous poisons

in the air, all destroy vitamins when breathed in by human beings. In self-defense, therefore, we must take extra vitamins every day, especially vitamins B and C, as these are known to aid in excreting poisons from the body.

As an example, pantothenic acid, one of the B vitamins, is known to detoxify the poisonous effect to streptomycin (*Science News Letter,* November 19, 1955). Streptomycin given alone can cause deafness, but this condition is prevented if vitamin B is given along with the streptomycin. It has also been shown that vitamin B can help to eliminate some of the DDT which is always accumulating in the body's tissues through what we eat. It also protects against the powerful poison, strychnine. It will neutralize the effects of the sulfa drugs, atabrine, and cortisone.

In two successive monthly circulars issued by Hoffman-La Roche, Ltd., a large drug firm (*Courier,* February and March, 1959), the subject covered is *Vitamins in the Treatment of Toxic Manifestations and Side Effects of Drugs.* Any doctor who reads the bulletins with their well-documented clinical test data, and then advises his patients to get their vitamins with their knives and forks, is not faithful to the best interest of these patients.

Older Persons Need More Vitamins

Older persons absolutely must take additional vitamins. As one gets older the little inner fire which is the body's metabolism begins to burn with a weaker flame, and the organs and glands become less efficient. One hears the expression that the circulation is slowing down. Under such conditions vitamin deficiencies are more apt to develop, because more vitamins are used to speed up the gradually failing metabolism. As we grow older, the process of aging causes us to develop nutritional needs which we did not have when we were younger. By taking extra vitamins we can prevent the senility which is bound to come under ordinary circumstances. It is not necessary to be half dead in our old age. There is medical evidence that the maintenance of the body's reserves of vitamins and minerals can prevent the deterioration of the eyes, ears, and hair and preserve the ability to walk without tottering and to think without doddering.

Then, of course, the doctor with his knife-and-fork theory does not consider people who eat all their meals in restaurants where additional chemicalizations are resorted to in the kitchen for various purposes. At least six situations exist there in which sodium chemicals are used.

Views of Some Authorities

One of the greatest nutritionists of our time, Dr. Henry C. Sherman, who was professor of chemistry at Columbia University, stated that vitamins A and C and calcium were the keys to longer life. He said, "Increase in the quantities of these 3 substances above levels commonly accepted as adequate have resulted in significant gains among laboratory animals. Clearly it is advantageous to the internal environment that the three nutrients be kept near the physiological saturation point."

Dr. Tom Spies of Birmingham conducted an experiment with 893 people who "had been old from the age of 30." These people, he said, were nutritionally disabled. Quoting *Cosmopolitan* (June, 1962): "He fed them diets rich in proteins, natural vitamins, and minerals, supercharged by doses of synthetic vitamins. To this he added quantities of dried brewer's yeast powder and liver extracts. The effects were almost miraculous. Forty-one of the men in the experiment were accepted for military service . . . Paul de Kruif, an ardent exponent of Spies' approach, points out that farmers feed their animals supercharged diets to keep them young and vital. Why not do the same for human beings? Dr. Edward J. Stieglitz, the great authority on aging, has noted that an optimum diet contains *five times* the protein and vitamins of the average minimum diet."

In view of what we have shown, how can doctors ask people to depend on their regular meals for their vitamins? How can doctors depend on the status quo of so-called balanced meals, when such "balanced" meals are leading to more sterility, more cancer, more heart disease, more mental trouble, and many other degenerative and other diseases? Do doctors reject vitamins because they don't have the facilities to test for them in the human body? What doctor has ever checked you for a vitamin deficiency?

This is exactly what Dr. Dorothy G. Wieble of the Milbank Memorial Fund said—the reason that nutritional deficiencies are allowed to go unchecked and unnoticed is that doctors don't know how to test for such deficiencies. But the American Medical Association continues to refer to vitamin-taking by the public as "Vitamania," and to the people who take them as hypochondriacs. It will be up to you after you read the chapters on specific vitamins in this book, to decide whether you will be a hypochondriac if you go on a program of taking extra vitamins.

7

Dr. Louis Berman— A Nutritional Blueprint

> *I will offer many orthodox medical scientists' work to prove that good nutrition and good mental power are directly related. Louis Berman, M.D. is one of these men. In other words, the system described in my book does not represent my own ideas. I have only been the one who has compiled many of them into one book—to weave them into a strong fabric, that, if adopted by you, can clothe you with greater mental and physical faculties than you now possess. Read and adopt!*

BEFORE WE launch into our discussion on individual vitamins, I would like to refer to a book written by Louis Berman, M.D. and published by Houghton Mifflin in 1932. It is called *Food and Character*. If you can obtain a copy of this book and read it, you will admit that Dr. Berman was a man who lived years before his time. More than 30 years ago he wrote that the chemistry of the brain will be found to be related to one's diet and to the endocrine gland secretions. One of the endocrine glands is the thyroid. He said, "The deliberate production of certified, chemically grade A brains will then come into prospect."

Dr. Berman, over 30 years ago, furnished a blueprint for mental health, but the medical people totally ignored his book and permitted psychiatry to take over—with a resultant steady increase in mental disease from year to year. Today over half the beds in hospitals are occupied by mental cases.

It would have been different if Dr. Berman was an excitable and emotional writer—but his book is a highly scientific volume, crowded with dozens of medical references to the work of many reputable research physicians and scientists. It is amazing also that in his book Dr. Berman states that the brain has a higher need for oxygen than any other organ of the body, because it has a higher rate of metabolism or using up of nutrients. This corroborates portions of our chapters on vitamin B, vitamin E, and exercise, which show how these things help to conserve the body's store of oxygen.

Vitamin B

Dr. Berman's thesis seems to rely strongly on the value of the B vitamins in maintaining and improving general mental health. Typical is an experiment he describes with two groups of rats in the observation of their ability to learn how to negotiate a maze. One group was nursed by mothers who had a vitamin B-rich diet. It took only 50 attempts for the vitamin B-rich group to learn the maze, whereas the others could not master it before 90 trials. Berman observes, therefore, that vitamin B is very important in the first few weeks of life when the brain is growing at a tremendous rate, and that it is important to give full feeding to babies in the first week especially, beginning with the first day. "It is quite possible," says Dr. Berman, "that *certain brains have been injured or made inferior* by poor feeding during the first few weeks of life."

Dr. Berman states that the brain is very rich in vitamin B, which is important to its efficient functioning because it builds the nerves. Injured nerves have been observed to be improved within three hours of the administration of vitamin B. A diet lacking in this vitamin may bring about a glandular instability, with a disturbance of the emotional balance. Many diseases of the nervous system are brought about by a lack of vitamin B in the body. Pellagra is one that involves the skin and the brain; in fact, insanity sometimes occurs in pellagra. In Egypt, says Dr. Berman, this is the chief form of insanity.

Berman describes an experiment at the Milledgeville State Hospital at Milledgeville, Georgia, with a woman epileptic, wherein it was discovered that vitamin B_6 (pyridoxine) is vital for the maintenance of the normal reactivity of the brain matter.

The Glands

Dr. Berman states that the quality of the diet affects one's emotional life by feeding the glands which have internal secretion. By means of these glands, there is a continual play upon the brain and the nervous system through which it acts. He says, "A certain amount of control of the destructive and ugly emotions fear, hate, and anxiety, can be attained through the regulation of food." There are chemical reactions in the brain caused by the action of the thyroid, adrenal, parathyroid and pituitary glands, but the operative efficiency of these glands depends on the quality of the body's food supply.

Berman relates Blanton's observations on 6,500 school children while in the army of occupation in Germany after World War I. Due to general malnutrition, he found them to be listless and apathetic. They tired easily. There was a decline in the standard of school work. There was more lisping and slurring of speech, and a rise in the number of mental defectives. There seemed to be a lack of nervous energy; the children could not concentrate; their memories were poor, and they were restless and irritable. It was due to a diet poor in proteins, fats, minerals, and vitamins.

He quotes from the work of Dr. Lydia Roberts, who was an authority on malnutrition in children. She said: "The rapidly developing brain and nervous systems of the child require certain essential food materials for normal growth. Moreover, the nerves need a moderate covering of fat to protect them from external stimulation. In a malnourished child, both of these conditions for a normal nervous system are apt to be lacking, the food materials more than likely being deficient and the nerves unprotected, owing to the lack of subcutaneous fat."

Weir Mitchell wrote a monograph called *Blood and Fat* as far back as 1891, describing how he treated nervous conditions by diets high in fat. The Sehams confirmed Mitchell's ideas. They found that by an adequate diet, symptoms of nervousness and irritability in children can be relieved. They then proved the same things by experiments on undernourished rats. To determine how nervous a rat was, they counted the number of times he blinked his eyes per minute. The undernourished rats blinked much more than the well-nourished ones.

Defective Diets Lead to Mental Inferiority

Cramer (quoted by Berman in a series of articles) said that one could produce mentally inferior children through defective feeding, and stated that many flunkers in school were starved for vitamins.

Berman tells an interesting anecdote about Sir Frederick Garland Hopkins, but since I found more information on it in Albert Von Haller's recent book *The Vitamin Hunters* (Chilton, Philadelphia), I will give that version:

"It had been noted in one of the large English boarding schools, that the pupils' achievements were declining to a remarkable degree, in sports as well as in their academic work. The boys became listless and irritable, many of them appeared sickly and in poor spirits. At first, the reason for the sudden change seemed quite incomprehensible. In this particular instance, responsibility rested on the shutting of a small fruit shop in the neighborhood of the school. Here the boys had been accustomed to spending their pocket money for fresh fruit. The supply of food in the school had been plentiful and quite in accord with traditional standards of the period, but there was practically no uncooked food such as lettuce, and the vegetables, as happens all too often when cooking is done for numbers of persons, were generally overcooked. The closing of the little fruit store had cut off the only source of vitamin C. Supplementary rations of fresh fruit in the diet of the boarding school soon restored the boys to their former state of health."

Schizophrenics Are Imbalanced Nutritionally

Dr. Berman himself, studying the diets of a series of schizophrenics (which includes *dementia praecox* and some other forms of insanity), found serious imbalances in their diets, especially with regard to minerals and vitamins. There was enough quantity but insufficient quality. He says that, "slight insufficiencies of the rarer minutiae of nutrition over a longer period of time," will produce breakdowns in weakened children who have come out unsatisfactorily from diphtheria, grippe, or scarlet fever.

He finds that the proper functioning of the endocrine glands is important in the prevention of this form of insanity, and states that physicians should concentrate on the correction of errors in diet, and thus correct the defects in these glands. Berman says further that practically nothing has been done to improve the oxygenation of the brain by special foods.

Berman discusses other forms of insanity, and winds up by saying that families with a history of this disease should eat large quantities of vitamins B and C. He suggests also the use of unsaturated fatty acids in generous quantities. Note that he said this over 30 years ago!

Dr. Berman states that it is not enough for the psychiatrist to use only analytic conversations and verbal education. There must also be an attack through the nutrition of the patient. But, on this latter point, we know that very little is done by psychiatrists.

The Brain Requires Good Nutrition

Berman states that the brain, in order to operate at its best, always needs certain kinds of food elements, especially during childhood when the brain is developing. "The human brain may be perfected by the control of diet sooner and more practically than by any of the other methods which have been proposed." He says that man has failed in becoming the master of his fate and the captain of his soul, because of lack of application of the knowledge of proper brain nutrition, and that although our so-called civilization and culture are contriving more inventions, in the midst of them there are increasing "deliriums, depressions, and hysterias, which are proof of the inadequacy of man's nervous system." He speaks about a threat to man's existence, a possibility of extinction in some terrible, large-scale catastrophe, the very suicide of man as a whole. Others have predicted this also. We are continually tampering with Nature. We are chemicalizing and fragmentizing. We are ignoring the basic importance of fundamentals while wasting scientific talent in attempting to conquer the stratosphere. As Thales observed (quoted by Aristotle)— while a star-gazer scanned the heavens, he did not see what was under his feet, and fell into a well.

Man is eating eggs laid by hens without benefit of roosters, and white bread with the living germ removed, restoring only part of the robbery with a few coal tar vitamins. Man is eating white rice, and potatoes without the skin—his nutritional history is a story of dozens of fragmentations. In the game of mental health, he is stacking the cards against himself!

A PROGRESS REVIEW

How to overcome the habits described in this book!

Up to this point we have urged you to be a meat-eater, to shun sugar, salt, tobacco, and alcohol, and to get yourself into the proper frame of mind to accept the fact that it is a healthy thing, in your search for greater mental ability, to take certain vitamins.

By this time you probably have made some attempt to put some of these ideas into action. I am sure that most of you have become aware that meat eating is important, and that you are taking enough of meat, fish, and eggs every day. These are easy things to take, unless you are a vegetarian. In that case there may be a problem. There are two kinds of vegetarians. One type does not eat meat because he believes it is not healthy to do so. There is some hope for him. The other forgos meat for humanitarian reasons —he thinks it cruel to slaughter animals for food. It will be almost impossible to influence him.

So what is the problem? If I were a vegetarian for a long time and I suddenly came across such a book as this I would start to reflect on my life during the vegetarian period. It is difficult for a person to assess his own mental status. I have seen what I consider "dumb" persons, who thought they were pretty smart. So I would try to figure it on the basis of my work. Have I lost jobs easily? Do I make very little progress at my jobs? If I were a teacher could I detect from my students' or superiors' attitudes towards me a recognition of mental ability or the opposite. I would try to be objective. Then if I feel that I am no Einstein, maybe I should give this Rodale guy's system a try! I wouldn't die if I ate meat for one year, would I? No you wouldn't unless you are hit by a truck or fall out of an airplane, or unless you are doomed to die because of a bad heart or some other organic weakness.

But even here I have news for you. The system described in this book will not only build a better mentality, it will also strengthen you physically in every organ of your body, so that your chances of dying of a heart attack will be far less than if you do not follow this system!

Well, let us go back to finding out how to force yourself to adopt the items in this program, brick by brick! Let us say you have solved the meat problem. You are eating plenty of meat every day and really savoring it. Now you wish to go further with the system. Next you are supposed to eliminate all white sugar from your diet!

Here I would like to describe something—a factor in getting people to be more health conscious which I think is very interesting. If you go to a certain type of person and say to him, "If you adopt these health measures you will live longer," he might laugh and say, "A short life and a merry one; what's a few years more or less if I have to give up such precious things? What? No ice cream? I'd rather be dead!"

But if I say to him, "If you adopt these measures you will become much more brilliant in your mental actions, you will do your job much better, people will look up to you, etc., etc., etc., and at the same time you will live a more healthy life and a longer one with a minimum of senility," I am sure that the most hardened offender would stop and listen, and perhaps be more easily sold on the proposition.

If you are having trouble with this system, then you should stop and do some special work to see how you can go about bolstering your will power generally! There are dozens of books on how to strengthen the will, which are full of tricks that show you how to accomplish things that you do not wish to accomplish. Every library is full of them.

Let me give you an example of a trick I am using this very moment in order to reduce weight. I have been on a weight reduction program, having reduced from about 179 down to 160 in the last 4½ months. I had wanted to get down to 155, but 160 was as far as my will-power would permit me to go. I would break away too often from my set "diet." So I figured out a trick. Here it was August 8, and my birthday is August 16. How about giving myself a birthday present of these five difficult pounds? It's a deal, I said, and set out to do it. In the next eight days I slowly fought my way through those five pounds. I don't think I would have accomplished it in any other way.

8

How Vitamin B Helps You Rise Above the Average

When you finish reading this chapter, the first thing you will ask yourself is, where can I get some extra vitamin B, other than what is in my diet, and secondly, how can I improve my diet so that there is more vitamin B in it! No matter how well you have been eating according to general popular medical opinion, you are only getting minimums, or at best averages, but averages will result in your being average mentally and physically.

But you want to get out of the average class! You want to put yourself in a special category, which you can positively do, if you read this chapter carefully and adopt its suggestions.

So FAR we have only been dabbling as far as nutrition is concerned. We have treated of the dangers of vegetarianism, sugar, and salt. But now I will bring up the heavy artillery and search in the interior of foods to see what they contain that is of importance to the health and functioning of the brain. We have already spoken of protein and carbohydrates, but now we come to vitamins, an altogether different animal. In my own definition, vitamins are sparks which help food elements to be properly absorbed and used in the body.

By and large, the group of B vitamins seems to be of greatest importance to the good health of the cerebral area. Vitamin B consists of many parts or fractions known as the vitamin B complex. Each part has many functions, but right now let us concentrate on the fact that, basically, vitamin B feeds the nerves and keeps them healthy, and since the actions of the mind are expressed through the nerves, where would we be mentally if our nerves were not in tip-top shape?

Now in our system we take many vitamins, but they must be of a natural, non-synthetic kind, which means that they are extracted from foods, not made of coal tar. In a later section of this book we will tell you why this is best over a long-term period. You can get vitamin B from wheat germ, tablets of brewers yeast, and desiccated liver. If you want to be in a high mental bracket, be sure that you take enough extra vitamin B every day. You can't get enough of it from your food.

Dr. Harrell's Work

Now let us see what the professionals have found with respect to the relationship of adequate vitamin B in the body to the health of the mind. Ruth Flinn Harrell, Ph.D., wrote a remarkable little book, *Effect of Added Thiamin on Learning*. Thiamin is one of the fractions of the vitamin B complex. The medical people prescribe these fractions separately, but if you take wheat germ, brewers yeast, and desiccated liver, you are getting the whole of the vitamin B complex, and don't have to worry about the parts.

At Johns Hopkins, Dr. Harrell cured a young man from aphasia—the loss of the power of expression by speech or writing—but didn't know exactly what was responsible for the cure. When they checked they found that vitamin B had been added to his diet. She experimented with several children who had never learned to speak because of a mental handicap. They learned much more rapidly when vitamin B complex was added to their diet!

Then she started a six-week project at the Presbyterian Orphans Home at Lynchburg, Virginia. Hundreds of children were involved, being divided into two groups, only one of which received added thiamin. In six weeks' time the thiamin group was superior in acuteness of hearing, and made measurably greater gains in learning ability. An infinitely small amount of this vitamin B fraction given over the ridiculously short period of six weeks had produced children who were superior both physically and mentally.

Another Experiment

In *The American Journal of Psychiatry* (Aug. '48), there is described an experiment with a small group of male patients at the State Hospital in Elgin, Illinois. They were given a diet very low in certain vitamins. After four to six months, "Mental abnormalities became much worse. One old man who had been quite amiable, became infuriated and threatened to break up the furniture and escape. A young man who had been subject to bad temper fits which ordinarily lasted a minute or so, once or twice a year, went into blind rages. These occurred in quick succession and lasted a half hour to an hour. During this time he would scream at the top of his lungs, throw heavy objects at anyone within reach and curse at the women attendants."

But as soon as their diets were supplemented with brewers yeast extract to give them the missing vitamin B, their symptoms dramatically cleared up. "The rage of the terrible-tempered old man subsided overnight and he became his former amiable self again. The young man who had endangered the lives of all around him appeared self-controlled the day after he was given the yeast extract. Only one old man took several weeks to regain his former contentedness."

In *The New York State Dental Journal* (1956, Page 319) there is an article commenting on an article in *The Journal of Psychology* as follows: "In contrast to psychogenic theories of mental illness, there is a growing amount of experimental evidence which indicates the possibility that some of the psychoneuroses and the functional psychoses are part of biochemical disorders of the body, and not illnesses of the mind as such. The original article presents a review of some of the experimental evidence, together with a discussion of some of its implications. Lack of thiamin at times results in ideas of persecution, mental confusion, and loss of memory; lack of riboflavin (one of the B vitamins) sometimes causes depression, visual disturbances, disorderly thinking, inability to concentrate or perform mental work, and forgetfulness; lack of niacin (another B vitamin) causes weakness, depression, anxiety, irritability, loss of memory, mania, hallucinations, and dementia (mental deterioration); lack of pyridoxine (B vitamin) causes epileptiform (epileptic) convulsions, general irritability, and weakness; in addition, lack of cyanocobalamin, biotin, and ascorbic acid (vitamins) are reported to cause similar types of mental disorders."

More Experiments

At the University of California, experiments reported in *The Archives of Pathology* indicated that a shortage of vitamin B_1 (thiamin) can cause extensive damage to the brain. Dr. James F. Rinehart, Dr. Louis G. Greenberg, and Melvin Friedman reported that monkeys whose diets were low in the vitamin showed a degeneration often involved in cases of palsy.

Here is a United Press item appearing in a recent newspaper, date not given:

"Ithaca, N.Y.—Scientists at Cornell University report that a lack of vitamin B_1 may play an important part in some mental illnesses.

"They say the vitamin, which is abundant in whole wheat, yeast, beans and liver, is important to the normal functioning of the brain."

In the Dec. 6, 1958 issue of *The Journal of the American Medical Association*, a case is described (quoted from *Nederl. Tidjdschr. Geneesk*, 102:1501-1503 (Aug. 2, 1958, Amsterdam) in which a 40-year-old woman was treated for severe depression. Electric shock treatments or chlorpromazine did not help. Chlorpromazine is a tranquilizer. When symptoms of pellagra occurred, she was found to be low in vitamin B (thiamin). They administered the whole vitamin B complex and it caused the complete disappearance of her psychiatric symptoms. Pellagra physically affects all the skin and tissues of the body and brings about general weakness.

Riboflavin

A shortage of another vitamin B complex fraction, riboflavin (vitamin B_2), can affect the mind. An anonymous psychiatrist writing in the July, 1954 *Atlantic Monthly* said, "In the southern states of the U.S.A., a group of persons became neurotic or mad in the spring of each year. They could only be encouraged psychologically to bear the apparently obvious precipitating burdens of poverty, poor food, and dismal homes. The discovery of vitamin B_2 now allows a simple drug to be given them which cures their mental symptoms despite their poverty and environmental stresses, until more vitamins become available to them in the growing crops."

Niacin

Another fraction of the B vitamins, niacin (Nicotinic acid) is an important factor in keeping us sane. I will cite a nine-year study at University Hospital, Saskatoon, reported in *The Lancet*, Feb. 10, 1962. They tried a half dozen cases early in 1952, the most dramatic being that of a boy of 17 admitted in February with acute schizophrenia.

"A few days earlier he had become excited, overactive, silly, deluded, and sometimes hallucinated. He improved briefly with electro-convulsive treatment, but subsequent insulin-coma treatment had to be stopped because of facial palsy. During the next three weeks his condition became much worse. Towards the end of May he was lying naked in bed, hallucinating, lalling incomprehensibly, urinating and defecating where he lay.

"Since we could do nothing else for him at this time, on May 28 we started him on five grammes of niacin with five grammes of ascorbic acid (vitamin C) daily, divided into four doses added to his tube-feeds. Next day tube-feeding was discontinued, and ten days later he was described as 'almost normal.' When he went home on July 21 his family said he was 'just as he'd always been.' He was still well five years later, and he has not been in a mental hospital since."

In September, 1952 in the same mental institution, there began a study with 30 patients from the psychiatric ward who were diagnosed as schizophrenic, the experiment lasting for 33 days. Of those who got the niacin (53), 49 became well. Of those who did not get niacin (23), only 11 became well.

Folic Acid

Regarding folic acid, another fraction of the vitamin B complex, the *Journal of Nutrition* of September, 1951, says, "Dietary deficiencies of many of the B vitamins are known to result in the degeneration of nerve tissue or the impairment of its function." It mentions seven researches performed at various institutions in which it was shown that mentality was affected by some factor in vitamin B. The article, by Whitley, O'Dell, and Hogan then proceeds to report the details of an experiment they conducted which showed that rats born to mothers fed a diet low in folic acid (one of the B fractions) produce offspring which if fed this same ration until near maturity are reduced in learning ability.

It is amazing how quickly the results of good nutrition can show itself. Recovery from apparent insanity within 15 minutes after a single dose of nicotinic acid, one of the fractions of vitamin B, was recently announced as an example of the spectacular achievements in conquering some forms of mental disease. The work was done by Dr. V. P. Sydenstricker and Dr. H. M. Cleckley of the University of Georgia, and was reported to the American Psychiatric Association.

Amazing Cure

The spectacular 15-minute recovery occurred in the case of a 66-year-old man who was admitted to the hospital in a greatly agitated state, not realizing where he was, and behaving irrationally. He shouted in broken sentences, tried to leap out of bed, and was constantly overactive and confused. The doctor's description is typical of the old idea of an insane person. While the nicotinic acid solution was still flowing into his vein, this man became quiet and co-operative, and within a few minutes showed no sign of his mental illness. This was not the action of a tranquilizer type of drug. It was from the effect of a vitamin.

Regarding the use of niacin for mental disease, there is a 161 page book devoted to it by A. Hoffer, M.D., a psychiatrist at the University of Saskatchewan. It is called, *Niacin Therapy in Psychiatry* (Charles C. Thomas Co., Springfield, Illinois). It describes many cases of the clearing up of various kinds of mental conditions by the use of that part of the vitamin B complex called niacin. Here is a typical case:

"Mr. P.B. was aged forty-seven. I first saw him standing naked in a sideroom on the 10th of February, 1952. He was very much afraid. Mr. P.B. was very talkative, overactive, and had numerous delusions and misinterpretations, all springing from a belief that "things had changed, looked strange, and were odd." He couldn't elaborate on this or explain what he meant. He was a short, thickset, well built, muscular man, inclined to drink a bit now and again. Not well educated. When he was well he had an outgoing and friendly disposition. He had only been ill for about seven weeks and had started by being depressed and withdrawn. In a general hospital, his behaviour had been seclusive and noisy. There was some uncertainty about his diagnosis, some believing that he had some brain damage; others that his was a schizo-affective illness.

"There were no signs of vitamin deficiency. In spite of sedation, he remained restless, was confused, but only for brief periods, refused to eat, and although stuporous at times, at others he was very overactive. On February 14th massive vitamin B treatment was started. This consisted of one gram of niacinamide daily plus small quantities of other vitamins. By February 16th he was much better, and next day he was out of seclusion and talking rationally. He remained on vitamins for some days, lost his fearfulness, and was well."

What interests me about the above book is that it has a chapter entitled, *Nicotine Acid as a Vaso-dilator,* meaning that it can open up the blood vessels. Niacin and nicotinic acid are the same drug, and the latter name has no connection with nicotine. But if such a tiny part of the vitamin total can be covered by a whole book with so many cases cured, you can imagine the magnitude of evidence that exists showing mental cases can be cured with vitamins.

An Expert Summarizes

For my money, the internationally famous nutrition authority, Dr. Tom Spies, sums up the subject very satisfactorily (*Journal of American Medical Association,* June 7, '58): "In patients with vitamin B deficiency and with mental symptoms, the cerebral metabolism was diminished by 60 percent."

Now, since the theme of this book is how to improve your mental ability, we shouldn't be bothering ourselves much with schizophrenia, aphasia, dementia, and general mental disorders. But I had to go into them a bit to show that a lack of vitamin B is the beginning of the path towards mental disease, and, while the average person never goes down the toboggan all the way, he may be touched to some extent, and suffer a partial loss in mental efficiency because of it.

So close the door to this possibility by being sure you are getting enough extra vitamin B through wheat germ, tablets of brewer's yeast, and desiccated liver. Make wheat germ flakes a part of your daily diet. Jars containing it are on sale at all groceries and supermarkets.

Also, of course, get vitamin B from your regular diet. The following is a list of foods that are abundant in this vitamin.

Beans:
    Lima
    Soy
Beef:
    Brain
    Heart
    Liver
    Steak
Brewer's Yeast
Cauliflower
Chicken
Eggs
Irish Potatoes
Lamb:
    Kidney
    Liver

Peas
Peanuts
Pork:
    Liver
Rice
Salmon (not canned)
Spinach
Wheat Germ Flakes
Beet Greens
Prunes, dried
Sunflower Seeds

Adequately supplied with this vitamin, in a few months you should begin to feel an upsurge in mental power, and see a better performance in connection with mental work you have to do.

REVIEW

Adequate meat, fish, eggs.

Low carbohydrate.

No sugar and salt.

No tobacco or alcohol.

Get enough vitamin B. Take wheat germ, tablets of brewer's yeast, and desiccated liver.

9

The Secret of Healthy Skin—Vitamin C

This chapter covers the importance of vitamin C in building brain power and mental energy. It is as simple as A, B, C, as well as D, E, F, K, and P. Vitamins are what give the electric spark to the digestion of your food, and cause more of the vital elements to be absorbed into the bloodstream to feed every organ of the body, including the brain.

Some doctors are against taking any vitamins other than what is in your food. Evidently they believe it is better for the world if people are only "average." They overlook the fact that it is mainly these "average people" who are involved in crime. You will also find that many of these "average people," by continuing whatever they are doing diet-wise, become vegetables.

So read, and then seek out a source of vitamin C.

VITAMIN C (the anti-scurvy vitamin) is basic to the health of the human body. It makes up a goodly portion of the *collagen*, or glue that holds the cells together. What can be more basic than that? One of the first things a vitamin C deficiency does is to affect the skin. Scurvy is an immediate effect of this deficiency. Because of such a condition, many people have a subclinical form of scurvy, which usually cannot be diagnosed, but which can affect the functioning of the body. Scurvy is merely the outside manifestation. What is affected inside is much more dangerous!

Vitamin C protects all the body tissues including the teeth, gums, bones, blood vessels, eyes, etc. It protects against infections and causes wounds to heal quickly. People who are low in vitamin C show bruise marks on slightest contact. But the most spectacular effect of over-doses of vitamin C is to prevent colds. Since this vitamin is water soluble, excesses do not accumulate in the body, but are excreted in the urine, perspiration, etc. Overdoses of vitamin C, therefore, are not dangerous.

Does vitamin C aid mental health in any way? Let us look into a few cases. Two doctors (E. H. Cranswick and T. C. Hall) conducted an experiment with 16 schizophrenics at Bunwell Hospital, in England, which was reported in *The Lancet* (March 25, 1950). Vitamin C was used, along with a hormone, deoxycortone. According to the doctors the treatment markedly improved all types of mental disorders, except the neuroses. According to *Science News Letter* (April 1, 1950), "Fourteen out of sixteen schizophrenics, depressives, and manics who had been sick less than one year became more rational and cheerful for a week after a single injection of the vitamin and hormone. After a series of injections, the improvement has persisted for three months so far." Mental disease, it seems, is a disease of things falling apart.

Science News Letter hails it as a chemical conquest. They should have called it a chemico-*dietetic* victory! To the public, the word chemical means drugs and medicines.

Mental Patients Are Low in Vitamin C

Long-time studies made on 173 patients in the Claybury Hospital, London, indicated that a large proportion of patients who had been in a mental hospital for long periods, had a low vitamin C status. This was reported in *The British Journal of Nutrition* (Vol. 6, No. 4, 1952). In the same hospital, another study indicated that the mental cases were lower in vitamins A and E than the private patients in the same hospital (*British Journal of Nutrition*, May 15, 1952).

The scandal of it is that mental patients were permitted to be in hospital for such long periods without correcting their vitamin deficiencies.

A very interesting letter written by a physician, regarding vitamin C and mentality, appeared in the May 12, 1962 issue of *The British Medical Journal*. It follows in part:

Sir, in 1953 Dr. H. Osmond and I began to treat some schizophrenic patients with large quantities of ascorbic acid (vitamin C), about 5 to 10 g. per day. It is my impression that the patients given ascorbic acid improved more quickly, but we conducted only single blind trials. One female patient, about age 45, was admitted with severe acute schizophrenia. The diagnosis was made by the chief of the service, who was not attached to the research. She also suffered from numerous secondaries from carcinoma of the breast. That day she was started on a regime of ascorbic acid—1 g. each hour, buffered with sodium bicarbonate. Forty-eight hours later she had received 45 g. and she was mentally well for six months, when she died from carcinomatous invasion. Certainly trials with ascorbic acid are indicated, but, as ascorbic acid is very rapidly excreted, large dosages should be given, at least 5 g. per day.

A. Hoffer.

University Hospital
Saskatoon, Saskatchewan.

Do you recognize this A. Hoffer? He is the same man who wrote the book on niacin we referred to in our last chapter. He seems to be involved in curing mental troubles with vitamins.

Schizophrenia Related to a Poor Diet

I will quote from another letter, signed by Gerald Milner, M.D., published in *The British Medical Journal* (Jan. 20, 1962):

In the annotation on malnutrition in old people (Dec. 2, 1962, p. 1486), you stressed the relationship of mental symptoms to malnutrition. Recently a chronic paranoid schizophrenic in this hospital developed gross self-induced dietetic scurvy. Throughout his six years as an inpatient, he has insisted on a diet of curried rice—and little else. . . . It required over 21 grams of ascorbic acid (vitamin C), given orally, to achieve saturation. His anemia recovered and his lesions (physical effects of disease on skin, etc.) resolved, as was to be expected, but his mental state underwent an impressive change for the better.

Despite heavy "tranquilization," he had always been "uncertain, disturbed, and aggressive". . . . Thorpe (*Journal Mental Science,* 1938, 84,788) found evidence of malnutrition in a significant proportion of admissions to a mental hospital, and Lucksch (*Wein, Klin, Aschr.* 1940, 53,109, and *Nutr. Abstr. Rev.* 1947, 17,505) noted considerable improvement in 12 schizophrenics given high doses of ascorbic acid.

One wonders how much vitamin C deficiency and malnutrition in general contribute to mental illness in the community (especially among old-age pensioners) and in chronic mental hospital patients.

Doctors Should Check Vitamin Status

The medical profession's disregard of the vitamin status of a patient's blood, which should be a routine test in all disease, is nothing short of a scandal. It is practically never done. In fact, the medical profession is continually hammering away on the theme of getting one's vitamins with one's knife and fork, and calls it a waste to spend money on vitamins. The whole concept of vitamins for health is pooh-poohed.

I have one more article on the subject of vitamin C. It was published in *The New Zealand Medical Journal* (April, 1962). It states that animals can be maintained in a condition of low mental health by keeping them low on vitamin C. It states further that in schizophrenia, early treatment to lower the blood copper and to increase the vitamin C should be of value.

It winds up by saying that disturbances in the vitamin C processes are commonly reported in schizophrenia, which results in "producing abnormal amounts of adrenaline metabolites, which may be the toxins of schizophrenia." We don't have to worry about those adrenaline metabolites, or know what they signify, but we can gather from this information that it is bad in schizophrenia cases to allow a deficiency in vitamin C.

Now what can we do about insuring ourselves against having an inadequate supply of this vitamin? We must oversaturate the body with it. We must shun daily minimums and double, triple, and even quadruple those amounts, because the excesses are eliminated from the body and the body must have much more than mere minimums. Secondly we must take vitamin C, not in the fragmentized ascorbic acid form, but in a whole natural form as in the rose-hip form of vitamin C, which also includes other vitamins and minerals. Rose hips are the little red berries which are the fruit of the rose plant. We want a "package deal," not a narrow artificially exact formula.

Vitamin C Destroyers

There are also things we do that destroy some of the body's vitamin C. Every puff at a cigarette or cigar destroys not a little vitamin C—the average heavy smoker is usually seriously deficient in this vitamin. A study should be made as to what percentage of people with nervous breakdowns are smokers.

Fruits and vegetables left unrefrigerated for several days may lose a lot of their vitamin C. Home canning of fruits and vegetables destroys vitamin C, for it is highly sensitive to heat and to air. Soaking vitamin C-rich foods or throwing away the water in which they are cooked is destructive of vitamin C. Cutting, slicing, grating, or chopping fruits or vegetables should be done just before they are eaten, for every cut surface exposed to air releases vitamin C. Baking soda in the cooking water or copper utensils destroy vitamin C instantly on contact.

Foods rich in vitamin C are:

Green peppers	Strawberries
Citrus fruits (we don't recommend)	Collards
Broccoli	Cantaloupe
Cauliflower	Turnip greens
Watercress	Tomatoes
Kohlrabi	Fresh peas
Raw cabbage	Potatoes

REVIEW

Plenty of meat, fish, and eggs.
Low starch consumption.
No sugar and salt.
No tobacco or alcohol.
Vitamin B—Wheat germ, brewer's yeast, desiccated liver.
Vitamin C—Rose hip tablets.

10

The Miracle of Vitamin E

Here you have the miracle vitamin—vitamin E. If you wish to encourage a free circulation of blood and its oxygen content to the brain, then vitamin E is for you. It will give you a free feeling all over the body, especially in the head.

Vitamin E has been known to keep diabetes in subjection, prevent heart attacks, save gangrenous legs from amputation, and build up the general health of the body. It assumes greater importance as the body ages, and can prevent senility and doddering of the brain.

Vitamin E is a must *in this system.*

IN STUDYING why we need extra vitamin E in our system of building mental power, we must think back to the chapters on salt and tobacco, in which we discussed the need to have sufficient width in our blood vessels to assure a good avenue of transport for oxygen. A lack of oxygen is involved in most cases of mental trouble. Vitamin E is an oxygen conserver and thus increases the oxygen available in the body. It also dilates the blood vessels—opens them up so that more oxygen can get through—from the toes to the top of one's head. For good mental health, good oxygenation is a *must*. D. D. Van Slyke, M.D., in the Bulletin of St. Francis Hospital and Sanatorium of January, 1957, said, "The brain is especially dependent on an uninterrupted supply of oxygen to maintain not only normal function, but organic existence. The adult human brain normally uses about 45 ml. of oxygen per minute. If the supply is cut down by 10 percent, one begins to get the first mental signs, a little difficulty in concentrating thoughts. If the oxygen supply is cut down by 20 percent, there results emotional instability and confusion; one might say it is equivalent in effect to three or four cocktails."

Experiments in High Blood Pressure and Diabetes

An article in an Italian medical journal describes an experiment in which 10 patients were treated with vitamin E for high blood pressure and diabetes. They showed an increase in mental clarity (*Policlinica-Sezione Prate.* 6, Terzani, 58, 1381-1951).

Drs. W. E. and E. V. Shute, in their book, *Alpha Tocopherol—Vitamin E,* talk of the help this vitamin can give to the aged who suffer commonly from the mental conditions (dementias) of arteriosclerosis. They state that about one-fifth of the persons with cerebral thrombosis go into mental breakdowns. "In the arteriosclerotic type," say these doctors, "the commonest symptoms are an apoplexy followed by characteristic mental changes, memory defects, occasional instability, outbursts of unreasonable anger. . . . Adequate nutrition is one of the most important points in adding life to the years if not years to the life. . . . The prevention of cerebral arteriosclerosis is the only real answer for this situation, and only alpha tocopherol (vitamin E) seems able to accomplish anything in this regard."

A doctor who has had much experience in treating mental cases with vitamin E is Alfonso del Giudice, M.D. of The National Institute of Public Health of Buenos Aires, Argentina. In an article in *The Summary* (June, 1960), a publication of The Shute Foundation, he said:

"Vitamin E (alpha tocopherol), a therapeutic agent still almost unknown in child psychiatry, opens up a wide horizon in the future for all mental insufficiencies and their consequences, by giving the therapeutist an instrument of extraordinary range. The secret of this normalizing action is based in the first place on massive doses, which do not act like small (vitamin) doses, but as therapeutic agents of pharmacological type; secondly on the stimulating effect of this agent on the neuro-hormonal system, which becomes evident only when the organism is saturated. . . ."

Helps Reduce Stammering

Dr. Giudice goes on to say that massive doses of vitamin E have reduced stammering and helped a great deal even in the most extreme cases, in which the spoken word is completely unintelligible. In his experience he has seen many disturbances of nervous and psychic origin greatly reduced by the administration of vitamin E. This includes the nocturnal terrors and fears of solitude of psychopathic children. At times, results are obtained in the incredibly short period of 11 or 12 days of treatment, in spite of the chronic nature of these disturbances, and the improvements achieved are permanent. Dr. Giudice has found that the tolerance for large doses of vitamin E is perfect and complete, even when taken in doses of two grams a day for years on end, as is his practice. This amounts to 2,000 milligrams or int. units of Vitamin E.

Dr. Giudice gave 20 case histories in a letter to *The Summary*. In each of them, mental disorder was effectively treated with vitamin E. It is not true that all of them were completely cured, but all were benefiting sufficiently so that the change was clinically observable.

We can see, therefore, how important it is that we have large amounts of vitamin E—far more than we can get from even a healthy diet. For best effect the body must be oversaturated with it. Vitamin E can be obtained either in drug or health food stores. Wheat germ contains some vitamin E, but not enough. But wheat germ *is* excellent for its vitamin B content.

The average bottle of vitamin E has a statement on it that one is to take one capsule a day of 100 milligrams. My wife and I have been taking 12 such capsules each day for many years. (We take the mixed tocopherols.) As Dr. Giudice has said, the secret of the effect of vitamin E lies in taking massive doses. The organism must be saturated.

REVIEW

Plenty of meat, fish, and eggs.

Low starch consumption.

No sugar or salt.

No tobacco or alcohol.

Vitamin B—Wheat germ, brewer's yeast, and desiccated liver.

Vitamin C—Rose hips tablets.

Vitamin E—I prefer the mixed tocopherols rather than alpha-tocopherol alone.

11

The Tonic That Helps You Feel Alive . . . Light Exercise

> *For optimum mental and physical efficiency you must exercise—a good brisk walk with a swinging gait one hour a day is "what the doctor ordered." It will tone up every organ and gland of the body, and give you a happier feeling. The mind jumps into spirited action when the body gets into regular movement.*
>
> *If you have been too sedentary, you have a wonderful treat in store for you! Keep moving as much as possible. Don't sit too long at a time— it depresses the mental activity!*

IT'S ABOUT time we took a breather from nutrition. While the title of this book indicates that we are studying the effects of nutrition on the mind, we can squeeze in the subject of exercise under a technicality; that is, exercise causes the digestive system to do a better job of digestion. Thus more nutriment is absorbed from the food—and the mind is better nourished. This is absolutely true! At any rate it is food and exercise—*both* of them—that make up the package. It is a package deal!

Exercise is a means of greatly contributing to the health of the body, and anything that improves the health improves the chances of the brain to function well. *Mens sana in corpore sano*—a healthy mind in a healthy body.

Years ago, when my son Robert was about 6 years old, he had a fear of riding in an automobile on long trips. He would get car sick. I would stop when I saw a long row of trees, and together we would walk under those trees. It never failed to put him into fine spirits, and we could resume the trip.

I have found that a good walk will always drive away melancholy. Researches have discovered that physical activity decreases nervous tensions. That is why white collar workers take more tranquilizers, sedatives, or pep pills than blue collar workers. Dr. Paul Dudley White in opening a gathering of cyclists said, "The best antidote for nervous tension and insomnia is some sort of physical fatigue. . . . If more of us exercised we'd have a sharp reduction in the amount of tranquilizers and sleeping pills in use today."

My Own Experience

I learned the value of exercise many years ago, when I thought that everything could be attained through nutrition. I found there was something lacking. I began to walk an hour every day, and soon discovered that this was the missing link. I noticed that it stimulated my thinking processes. I have a habit of making notes of ideas that come to me no matter where I am. Soon I was averaging about 20 written notes in an average one hour walk. I learned to write my notes while walking. Later I invited my attorney to walk with me when he had business to discuss. In writing plays, when I reach a situation where I am unable to go further, I go for a walk, and ideas come tumbling out of my mind, one after another. Some of the best twists in the plots for my plays have come while walking.

Professor George L. Cunningham of Cedar Crest College (Allentown, Pa.), who owns over 300 patents centering around producing chemicals industrially, and who was instrumental in developing some of the original high-energy fuels for space rockets, claims that he does most of the work in his head—while taking a walk. Evidently exercise stimulates all the glands of the body, making them function more actively and causing them to secrete their glandular substances, hormones, etc. Exercise stimulates *all* the processes of the body. The swinging gait of a walk is one of the finest mental stimulants. Exercise increases the oxygenation of all the tissues of the body including those of the brain, and we have seen how important this can be.

Another Example

Here is an item from *The Canadian Medical Association Journal* (1:265, March, 1911), that shows the value of exercise:

"Among university students it has been demonstrated that an appreciable acceleration in growth and weight can be produced by carefully supervised exercise, and this is accompanied by an increase in mental efficiency. The hunger for muscular exercise natural in all growing children and young men must be stimulated and satisfied if their efficiency is to be safeguarded, and no medical education which ignores this problem can lay just claim to completeness. Dr. Tait McKenzie, while he remained in Canada, taught this lesson incessantly, and he has continued to teach it in the United States from his chair in the University of Pennsylvania."

Note in the above quotation the increase in mental efficiency due to exercise.

A simple thing like daily walking is one of the finest preventatives of senility. People who do not walk enough every day, for example, develop swelling at the ankles, which is a form of senility. When we use our legs, their muscles expand and contract, causing the lymphatic process in the legs to function efficiently. Otherwise, there is a defective lymphatic circulation, and it is then easy for gravitation to cause the lymph to move down to the ankles and cause *edema*, or swelling, there. Sufficient daily walking will enable one to go into old age with the slender graceful ankles that are not associated with tottering. But the important thing is that the condition just described can slow down the general circulation which can affect other parts of the body, including the mind.

Several Other Cases

Here is a case described in the *Canadian Medical Association Journal* (July 30, 1960), which gives more evidence. I will quote:

Case 1. An 81-year-old fisherman fell in his boat and suffered a fracture of his femur. The hip was pinned twice, the first attempt being unsuccessful. He had typical generalized arteriosclerosis, with mild arteriosclerotic brain disease. He had a poor memory for recent events and was emotionally unstable. With inactivity, his mental condition deteriorated, and he became quite childish. However, as soon as he could walk he went fishing again alone, despite continuing hip pain. His catch was about 1000 pounds of fish a week. His mental status improved greatly.

Case 2. A fisherman, aged 78, underwent throughout one winter progressive depression and withdrawal. He was visited for an attack of broncho-pneumonia, and this gave the opportunity for continuing treatment with a high-vitamin diet and simple supportive psycho-therapy. He improved on this, but as soon as the better weather came and he was able to return to fishing, he became once more the cheerful old man he had been previously, and maintained this status throughout the next winter with elementary support.

Many of these old men grew up in the days of oar and sail, and are remarkably healthy. The process of natural selection in that era is probably responsible for part of this, for men who were not suited to fishing, either physically or mentally, would tend to leave the island to work elsewhere. But it is interesting to note that Weir, who was physician in the islands for 26 years, points out that in a population of 2000 he saw only six cases of myocardial infarction (heart attack) among men under 70 during that time, and those six cases were in men leading sedentary lives. The tremendous physical exertion of hauling a trawl or lobster-traps by hand continued until quite recently, so that even the middle-aged group were exposed to this in their youth.

Hill Walking Best

Quite some time ago I discovered that I was in better physical shape when my walking was in hilly land, rather than on the flat. This was confirmed by the experience of Konrad Adenauer, former Chancellor of Germany, who is nearly 90 years old and ticking on all mental as well as physical cylinders. He was recently interviewed by a delegation of West German sports writers who asked him for his formula. "Two things," replied Adenauer. "One is the Italian game of *bocce,* which I indulge in as often as possible. Secondly, I have been living at Rhondorf, where

I can only get home by climbing up the path. It is more than 50 steps, another advantage of the hillside location; the villa—although one of the finest in the whole Rhine Valley—was not appropriated by Occupation officers after World War II, because they could not drive up to the door in their cars."

Years ago I read an interview with an old Armenian living in New York City who was 115 years old, who was in possession of all his faculties. What was the cause of his longevity and cheerful frame of mind? The old man claimed that for many years he walked practically all day long, stopping to chat with friends, and sitting down occasionally to rest or to eat.

An item in *Today's Health* (June, 1960), describes some research done at the University of California which proved that regular physical exercise greatly increased a person's sense of well-being, and that it boosted his ability in taking nervous strains, disappointments, and frustrations. There were two groups, only one of which was given supervised exercise. This group's morale was higher and they developed an ability to adjust to nervous stress. It was found that exercise releases nervous tensions. Walking and swimming were highly recommended.

For maximum results I suggest doing calisthenics as well as walking—not more than 5 to 15 minutes a day. Between this and a walk of at least an hour a day, you will be doing a great deal to further the effect of your nutritional program to improve the health and well-being of your mind. Don't say you don't have the time—squeeze the time in anyhow! You will find that your other work will get done somehow. In fact, the exercise will enable you to do your other work in less time! And don't be afraid to walk in a big city. Vitamins B and C will enable your body to excrete much of the pollution poisons you breathe in.

So remember—for a better functioning mind you must walk an hour a day.

12

You Are What You Eat—
The General Diet

> *It has been an old medical adage, known even in primitive times, that you are what you eat. What you eat today, thinks tomorrow! You can study all you want, but if your diet is not correct, yours will not be a first rate brain, insofar as its maximum action is concerned.*
>
> *In your new methodology, to help your brain to improve in its general efficiency, look to your diet! Learn what you must leave out and what you must add to it. Start at once! But you need not adopt the suggestions given in this chapter all at once. Consider which one you wish to start with, and gradually, adopt them all one at a time.*

WE HAVE discussed, individually, protein, carbohydrates, various vitamins, food items like salt and sugar, and a few other things. Now let's put some time in on the effect of the general diet on the mind, because to really develop to the maximum your ability to work with your mind, everything you eat will have to be given the closest scrutiny.

This can be seen in research work done with high school students in various parts of our country. Students at South Houston High School in Texas were not doing too well in their studies. They were found to be eating terrible breakfasts—sugared soft drinks, potato chips, a cup of coffee (with sugar), a biscuit, and a nerve pill—sometimes a vitamin pill (synthetic variety). They went through a nine-week experiment, eating breakfast and lunch at school, their evening meal prepared by their parents as specified by the school. They ate a well-balanced diet, based on modern ideas of nutrition. It resulted in an improvement in the grades by 44 percent of the participants.

According to the *Journal of Psychology* (45:47-74, 1958), where school boys omitted breakfast for a two-week period, there were detrimental effects on their scholastic attitudes and attainments.

In an article in *The Journal of the American Medical Association* (Nov. 1, 1941), Dr. Norman Jolliffe discusses the subject of curing neuro-psychiatric disorders through nutrition, and advises that the diet contain as much as possible of natural, unrefined foods. He suggests that the following be excluded: sugar, candy, jellies, jams, white flour products, refined cereals, polished rice, and alcoholic drinks.

A Louisiana Example

In 1943, in a Louisiana parish (county) called Ascension, the problem of poor efficiency in classwork was becoming acute. The scholastic rating of the parish's schools was embarrassingly below the national average. A whole new approach to the problem was taken here when it was found that the dietary habits of the children who attended school were also appallingly bad. A survey disclosed that 1 percent of the 2,500 school children concerned ate what would be called a "good diet." Over 33 percent ate what had to be called an actually "poor diet." Then a change took place. The school superintendent inaugurated a program aimed at making everyone—children *and* parents— diet conscious. Perseverance made the program a success, and the proper eating habits of the pupils soared. With the improved nutrition came a miraculous increase in scholastic accomplishment. By 1950, the parish was well above the national average in the rating of its students' learning ability (*The Sign*, February, 1952).

In an item in *The Medical Press* (245:2:30-34), Dr. G. H. Collins of Kingsway Hospital in Derby, England, says that mental fatigue is often partly based on long-standing defects in the diet. He states, "Attention to the nutritional habits of children and adults may prevent disorders of mental health developing later. In all psychiatric disorders, from the behavior disorders of childhood to the chronic deterioration of senile psychoses, faulty nutrition may play a role."

Here is an item from *The St. Petersburg Times* (Oct. 24, 1961):

" 'Poor nutrition may be the cause of some bad grades in school,' according to Dr. George M. Cummins Jr. of Northwestern University. 'Bad eating habits can lead to physical and emotional problems that can impair scholastic performance,' he said."

A teacher, Mrs. Marjorie Auwater of Millington, Michigan, is quoted in the *New York Times* of Jan. 4, 1955 as saying that classroom indifference may be due not to laziness but to diet. She made a study of 73 teen-age girls and found that 24 of them ate only one meal a day consisting of candy bars, soda, peanuts, french fried potatoes, or cookies.

Diet and Insanity

"Can a poor diet cause insanity?" This question begins a news item in the *San Francisco News* (May 6, 1957). It answers with the following:

"The question has been answered by Dr. Charles L. Yeager, who believes lack of proper food may induce mental disturbances. He produced evidence to support the old German maxim, 'One is what one eats,' at a conference of the aged at the Women's Club of San Francisco. He was one of more than 200 specialists of the Western Gerontological Society who discussed progress in their field.

"Tests are under way, he said, to indicate that older persons often turn unaccountably to sweets and less nourishing foods. Their families believe they are being well nourished, he said; nevertheless, they lack adequate proteins, minerals and vitamins. The deficiency may cause chemical changes in the brain, the physician suggested, and these are strongly related to the confusion and loss of memory associated with age. He said senile psychotics at Napa State Hospital improved steadily when their diets were enriched."

At the National Animal Disease Laboratory at Ames, Iowa, they reversed the personalities of ferrets by improving their diet. The ferret is a wanton killer of poultry, has been known to attack children, and normally exhibits no affection, even for its master. The female, at times devours her young.

A group of ferrets recently arrived at the laboratory at Ames. They were so difficult to handle that their caretakers had to wear heavy leather gloves for protection. But after being fed a diet of three parts of fresh horse meat, two of dog meal, and one of fresh milk, their characters changed and they could be cared for without gloves.

In a Russian research *Voprosy Pitaniya* (Vol. 21-1962), experiments showed that a high carbohydrate diet (in animals) increases their excitability, while a high-protein diet depresses it. The continuously rising consumption of sugar must have some bearing on the increasing excitability of the people of our times.

I think you have had enough evidence to convince you that there *is* a relation between a good diet and a good mind. But now let us go off on a bizarre tangent.

Sick Moose

I was startled to read in the February 19, 1954, issue of the *New York Times* the following:

> *Ottawa, February 16*—Canadian biologists are studying herds of mentally sick Nova Scotia moose in the hope of learning something about the treatment of human madness. About half of the moose in the province are believed to be out of their minds as the result, it is thought, of the physical deterioration of their brains caused by malnutrition.
>
> Researches by the provincial Lands and Forestry Department so far lead the biologists to conclude that the climatic changes that have taken place in Canada during the last few hundred years lie behind the moose madness.
>
> As the climate grew warmer, certain types of plant food on which the moose depended for a balanced diet disappeared. Normally, the moose would have moved north in search of cooler temperatures and essential foods, as they have in other parts of Canada. But Nova Scotia is a peninsula, with a narrow land-bridge to the mainland, and the moose are hemmed in.
>
> As a result they are slowly dying of malnutrition. Scrawny and tick-infested, they lope around the countryside, their motor and sensory nerves out of order. Half blind, they crash into fences or get entangled in bushes and trees until they die.

Biologists are attempting to treat the moose by feeding them the minerals that are believed to be 'acking in their diet, much in the way Nova Scotia farmers give their cattle supplementary cobalt to keep them well.

The researches hope soon to have proof that the brain disease from which the moose are suffering is caused by a dietary deficiency of certain minerals and vitamins. Once such proof is established, they say, ways may be found of curing or alleviating human mental disorders by means of a corrective diet.

I don't know what the status of those moose are today, but it would be interesting to find out. This would make a pleasant excursion for some psychiatrists with time on their hands, or who are in need of a vacation.

A Visit to Central America

Some years ago during a visit to Central America, I noted a peculiar fact about the dogs there. I don't think I heard one of them barking or being angry. They seemed rather quiet, with an air of general lethargy about them. They didn't look dynamic! I associated it at the time with something about their diet. There is so much poverty in that region that probably the dogs are not getting enough high class protein. It is a case, I am sure, where the diet has affected the character of the animals, and it could involve the functioning of the brain. So here is another excursion trip for a group of psychiatrists who would take some nutritionists and biochemists along with them.

I would like to speak about something that is happening to chickens that are kept under commercial conditions and fed with synthetic modern chicken feeds. According to *The Akron Beacon Journal* (April 6, 1961), there is bedlam in the hencoops. Thousands of chickens in Medina County, Ohio have gone stark, raving mad. "The hysterical birds emit terrible shrieks, flap and panic and sometimes pile up and smother themselves, with losses running up to thousands of dollars."

The farmers have tried feeding them tranquilizers with no result. "One poultryman hoses down his flock with water to quiet them." The hens eat twice as much feed and still remain skin and bones, and a flock that should be laying hundreds of eggs a day will lay only seven or eight. The chicken feed is changed but nothing helps. Experts from all over the country, including poultry psychiatrists, have moved in but can't seem to pinpoint the trouble. But let's look at the chickens on our farm. We have had three to four hundred at all times for the last 20 years, who have been fed a healthy diet, and who are perfectly stabilized both mentally and physically. I can walk into the chicken loft, and there will not be the usual pandemonium which occurs at other farmers' chicken lofts when I visit there.

The other day I was walking along a country highway, and passed a neighbor's chicken house. There was a high window at which about six of his chickens were roosting. When they heard my footsteps they flew off the roosts with a great nervous clamor. From my experience I know that these chickens are getting the regular commercial feeds which evidently are lacking in some nutritional elements.

Now people are the same as moose, dogs, or chickens, in that if they are not fed properly it could affect them mentally. If they eat the regular supermarket groceries without supplementing them with natural vitamins and minerals, if they eat a diet low in protein and high in starch and sugar, they are bound to get so that they "fly off the roost" at the slightest provocation.

A Letter

I would like to present a letter from one of the readers of *Prevention*. I am not presenting it as something scientific, but I feel that it *is* significant to the theme of this book. It comes from Mrs. Don Blaylock of Winston, Oregon:

"My husband and I were both falling apart at the seams when we were introduced to *Prevention*. I had racked up a total of two nervous (mental) breakdowns and my husband was currently saddled with an ulcer of the duodenum. We started throwing out the bella donna and phena-barbitol my husband was taking (doctor's orders), and I said goodbye to the Thorazine and Equinel tranquilizers I had been gulping for quite some time.

"I know now that my illness was caused from severe nutritional deficiencies, and those were just about every one in the book, but particularly the B vitamins. Emotional upsets and stresses and frustrations do contribute to mental illness, but I find that with an adequate diet I am able to face these things and endure more and accept them much better and work them out sensibly and practically

"I've also learned about sugar—or anything containing sugar. Shortly after eating sweets I became extremely nervous and irritable and upset. If I've eaten quite a lot of sweets I feel almost frantic, or a sort of frenzied feeling. Coffee gives the same type of reaction but not so severely.

"Have found that whole wheat bread or any wheat products disagree with me. About an hour or two after eating wheat products an overwhelming feeling of fatigue sets in—and a very uncomfortable or sickish feeling in my stomach. Oatmeal mush reacts the same way. I have learned that eating as many raw fruits and vegetables as I can gives me the best degree of health. I never thought I would see the day, but cooked foods are beginning to seem a little repulsive to me at times. Of course we both take the natural food supplements in addition to our other foods.

"My husband's ulcer no longer bothers him, so it would seem it has healed. We discovered that flaxseed meal and olive oil mixed together and taken every day and cabbage juice are extremely valuable for ulcers of the stomach or duodenum."

We must bear in mind that the brain is not a finished product. The blood is continually nourishing it. All cells in the body, wherever they may be, are in a cycle of destruction and rebirth. Old ones die—new ones take their place. Recent research by atomic scientists has revealed that over 98 percent of the body is renewed every year, including the brain. The organs are renewed through circulating blood and any child should know that there is a vast world of difference between the blood chemistry of a well-nourished and an ill-nourished person.

REVIEW

Plenty of meat, fish, and eggs.
Low starch consumption.
No sugar or salt.
No tobacco or alcohol.
Vitamin B—wheat germ, brewer's yeast, and desiccated liver.
Vitamin C—Rose hip tablets.
Vitamin E—the mixed tocopherols in heavy dosage.
Exercise—calisthenics and walking.
No refined foods.
   If you're doing all these things you should begin to feel a clearer and a more energized mind!

13

The Danger of Chemicals in Our Food

> *This chapter will show you the dangerous effect of certain types of toxic chemicals that are added to our foods, and the liquids we ingest every day which weaken the body and the mind. It will give you a simple rule, which, if followed, will reduce these chemicals to a minimum.*
>
> *Read the small print on all packaged food items, and if the substances mentioned are chemicals such as propionates, monostearates, glycerides, etc., leave them alone.*
>
> *The less such chemicals are in your diet, the less interference there will be with the ability of your mind to act positively!*

CERTAIN FOODS we eat are detrimental to our mental health, but there is yet another thing about foods in general that we have to be careful about, and that is the chemical additives that are used in the manufacture of food products for various reasons. What is the effect of these chemicals on the functioning of the mind? Most of these chemical additives are toxic substances, or poisons. True, they are used in such tiny quantities that they do not kill—at least, not at once. But there is the effect of a host of different additives which you consume from morning to night, including the chlorine and aluminum sulphate in drinking water, which all add up.

I am certain that these toxic chemical additives have a deleterious effect on the functioning of the human mind. A clue may be the fact that poisons were recently shown to be a cause of dreaming. Freud has said that dreams stem from psychological needs of the dreamer to release various unconscious thoughts and emotions in his sleep. Freud overlooked the chemical cause of dreams.

Dr. William C. Dement, a world authority on sleep and dreams, and a neuro-physiologist in the department of psychiatry at Stanford University, has found that dreams are part of the body's efforts to clear the nervous system of poisons. He proved this with cats and with 17 humans. He refers to his "poisons" as a naturally created "toxin" from the central nervous system, but I wonder whether he can be sure of that point. What would be the difference between the action of a naturally created poison, or a poison that found its way into the nervous system through the food?

Bread Chemical Gives Fits to Dogs

Years ago, nitrogen trichloride was used to bleach white flour, but when fed to dogs in an experiment in England, by Sir Edward Mallanby, it gave them running fits. What effect does nitrogen trichloride have on the mind of man? In commenting on the effect of ingesting nitrogen trichloride, Sir Edward said, "We certainly have enough chronic degenerative diseases of the nervous system of unknown (cause) to suggest that this matter is worthy of consideration."

Nitrogen trichloride in bread has been banned and chlorine dioxide substituted as a flour bleach, but when bread so treated was fed to mice, it slowed down their growth. This probably indicated that it slowed down *every* process in the body. Is it possible that the thinking ability of a person consuming such bread will be slowed down?

All toxic chemicals are bound to come in contact with the nerves of the body, including those in the brain, thus reducing their functioning ability. A toxic chemical taken into the body is like a wild animal set loose in the streets of a city.

The worst chemicalizations occur in the making of breads and cakes. The late Lord Addison defined baking as "the art of making water stand up," and this is done with all manner of added chemicals.

A Washington physician, Dr. Eloise W. Kailin, working with three patients, found that many Americans may be suffering from intolerance to food stored in plastic containers. Toxic chemicals from the plastic substances get into the food which is in contact with it, and, in Dr. Kailin's opinion, can cause emotional depression and mental confusion.

In recent psychiatric studies, analyses of the blood have shown toxic chemicals to be present in patients with mental disease, but nothing is said about the fact that these chemicals could come from the additives used in foods.

Chemical Poisoning of the Brain

Dr. Howard Fabing, Cincinnati psychiatrist, believes that "mental illness could be caused by chemical poisoning of the brain, rather than being something we worry or fret ourselves into."

In Bicknell's book *Chemicals in Food*, he has an entire chapter called "The Prevention of Diseases of the Nervous System." I will go down the line and give a few ideas from it: A patient who has developed a nervous disease may be better off by avoiding heavily chemicalized margarine. (Margarine can contain benzoate of soda, butylated hydroxyanisole, monoisopropyl citrate, yellow coal tar dye, Diacetyl as a flavorer, Stearyl citrate as a metal scavenger, etc.)

In connection with certain diseases that affect the mind, Parkinsonism, Paralysis Agitans, or the Shaking Palsy, "it would seem wise for patients to avoid foods possibly contaminated with any of the chemicals which damage the nervous system—lead, mercury, and many of the agricultural insecticides, and indirectly, the emulsifiers used in commercial cooking which may cause the bowel to absorb into the body toxic substances that are normally voided."

Did you know that (to prevent melting) ice-cream, cheeses, margarine, and other foods are just loaded with these emulsifiers? These can unquestionably damage the nervous system, and bring about a malfunctioning of the brain system.

In Iowa a few years ago, there were cases in which children's faces and ears turned red and itchy after eating hamburger. Hamburgers and hot dogs are treated with sodium nitrite, a most toxic substance used to preserve the meat and make it look fresher in the store. Faces turning red are only an outward sign of damage. We cannot see the brain tissues and nerves turning color, but this may actually take place.

We also must not overlook the effect of insecticides. Rachel Carson in her book *Silent Spring,* brought evidence to prove that there is a direct connection beween the use of insecticides and mental disease. Miss Carson said that according to medical research, Lindane is stored in significant amounts in the brain and liver tissue and may induce profound changes in the central nervous system. Yet this compound is much used in devices that pour a stream of volatized insecticide vapor into homes, offices, and restaurants.

The brain is about the most delicate organ in the body and depends on the health of the whole body to keep it going. The toxic substances, food additives, and insecticide residues on fruits and vegetables destroy vitamins, combine with and inactivate minerals, and destroy enzymes (which are extremely delicate substances) which partake in all body processes including the functioning of the brain. If you can realize to what extent your food is chemicalized, it should frighten you into going on a program to beat the chemical system. You must understand that these chemicalizations are not done to protect you, but to gain more profits for the food producers.

Plan to Avoid Chemicals

I have found a way to beat this system. I eat no foods made in a factory. This leaves out bread, cakes, butter, cheese, boxed cereals, all packaged and canned goods—no candy, sodas, ice-cream, etc.

Do you think I am starving? Hardly! I can eat to satiety of the following:

MEATS—but only fresh meats. No processed hot dogs, smoked and salted meats, no salamis, pastramis, bolognas, etc.

FISH—only fresh fish—no smoked or preserved varieties; but only seagoing fish. Inland waters usually are polluted.

EGGS—two eggs a day.

FRUITS—fresh fruits.

VEGETABLES—fresh and frozen vegetables.

For bread I have substituted corn pancakes made with eggs, wheatgerm flakes, blackstrap molasses, and the whole ground corn. Beware of the de-germinated corn flour on the market!

And watch for the small print on the packaged food! On packages of figs, dates, etc., look to see that they have not been sulphur treated.

Also: Since we are living in a chemicalized world you are bound to breathe in air pollutions, and will take in some pesticide chemicals with the fruit and vegetables you consume. To counteract this be sure you are taking enough of vitamins B and C, brewer's yeast, wheatgerm, desiccated liver, and rose hips. These aid the body in excreting poisons.

And if you work in a gasoline station, or a factory where toxic chemicals are manufactured, either change your job or increase the amounts of vitamins B and C you take. In fact, in such case go very strong on the system described in this book, and do plenty of walking in the open air.

A Plan to Limit the Amount of Chemical Additives You Consume

If you will adopt my idea of eating no foods made in a factory, with a few safe exceptions like packaged raisins, etc., you will already have eliminated a tremendous percentage of additive chemicals you have been consuming up to now. You will have stopped eating cheeses and other dairy products. Cheeses not only contain emulsifiers and other chemicals, but they are also heavily loaded with salt. Also, do not drink milk, as it is made in a factory—for what is a cow if not a factory, the way they have over-bred her? Besides, milk contains residues of DDT, penicillin, often hydrogen peroxide (as a bacteria killer), oat gum (as an antioxident), and sometimes other chemicals as well.

The remaining categories of foods that are chemically tainted are the fruits and vegetables that have been sprayed with poisonous insecticides, and don't think that if you cut off the skins, you are avoiding these poisons, because they are usually absorbed into the interior of the fruit. The problem here is to see how much we can cut out in these two categories to cut our insecticide consumption to a low level.

As between apples and pears, the latter receive far less insecticide than the former. Therefore, cut out apples entirely, and eat pears only occasionally, if at all. If you buy in health food stores, you can get raisins, figs, and dates that are pretty safe.

Nuts

This is rather a large group, and a very healthy one. Their hard shells protect them from poison sprays of all kinds. Walnut, brazil nut, hazel nut, filbert, Indian or

Pinyon nuts, and also peanuts and chestnuts. The peanut grows underground and therefore is doubly protected. I knew a man who lived to be over 90, and in his last 30 years he lived almost exclusively on nuts.

Do not buy shelled nuts. They are cheaper and healthier if purchased in their shells. In the factories, chemicals are sometimes used to shell nuts.

Coconut

Another food protected by a heavy shell is the coconut, which is rich in minerals. In many warm countries it forms the main staple of the diet.

Pineapple

Should not be the canned variety. Its heavy skin protects this fruit from poisonous insecticides that seep through the skins of other fruits. The pineapple is very rich in vitamin C, protein, and enzymes which aid digestion.

Watermelon, Honeydew, Cantaloupe

All are protected by heavy skins and are excellent foods. We scoop some of the inside pulps of the cantaloupe, along with the seeds, and break it up in a blender to make a very satisfying and nutritious drink. The seeds are a very potent item of nutrition.

Avocado

It has a thick, dark green skin, with a meaty melon-like pulp, and is known to be a very healthy food.

Pumpkin and Squash

Can be served mashed (as are turnips or potatoes), or it can be cubed and boiled. Europeans enjoy pumpkin soup. It can be mixed in a blender to make drinks of various kinds.

Potatoes

Both white and sweet potatoes grow underground where they do not receive direct applications of insecticides. I highly recommend sweet potatoes. Potatoes are not half as fattening as bread and cake.

Beets and Carrots

Both grow underground and are a desirable addition to your diet.

Eggplant

Its thick skin repels many dangerous chemicals. It is rich in vitamins A and C.

Peas and Beans

These are protected by their pods.

Radishes, Turnips, Parsnips

All grow underground, and are not directly sprayed.

Wild Rice, Brown Rice, Corn

The corn is well protected by its sheath, the wild rice grows under natural conditions, and brown rice has had a minimum of chemical contacts.

Sunflower and Pumpkin Seeds

These two seeds happen to be a most marvelous food, and are well protected from chemicals. For anyone aiming at developing the highest degree of health, these seeds are strongly recommended. The seed is a live food. When planted in the soil, an enormous amount of plant tissue will grow out of it. It therefore contains rare minerals, vitamins, and life-giving substances that are highly desirable for optimum nutrition. They can be obtained shelled, or hulled for easy eating, in all health food stores.

Olive and Other Oils

Olive oil, a tablespoonful at each meal, will keep a stomach ulcer under control, and is a worthwhile item of diet for general health. The olive tree lives for thousands of years. There may be something in the sap that promotes health and longevity. The Italians thrive on it.

Of course, you may not want to stick 100 percent with these foods. But with regard to others, moderation is the word, and you will in time feel the benefits of a diet very low in chemical additives.

You will of course add to the above—fresh meats, fish, and eggs.

14

How to Keep Your Driving Record Clean

> This chapter may be the means of saving your life, by preventing you from getting into an automobile accident. If you follow the system described in this book, your mind will have a sharper edge. It will be able to make split-second decisions in an emergency.
>
> In fact, if this book can reach enough people and get them to adopt its suggestions, then when you have a close call with another car, wouldn't it be something if the driver happened to have read this book, and changed his dietetic ways? Then both of you could maneuver quickly without your cars colliding!
>
> The general level of automobile accidents can decline if the nutrition of the country in general can be improved. So, after you have read this book, turn it over to another person. Or, better yet, give it as gifts to some of your friends, employees, or business associates.

ONE OF THE extra dividends you will get if you follow our entire system is that you might *not* be maimed or killed in an automobile accident. The ability to make a quick emergency decision at the wheel may depend on your store of mental energy, or on whether you are adequately equipped with vitamins.

A piece of German research was written up in *The Boston Herald* of June 12, 1957. A group of 152 problem drivers in Germany were given 150,000 units of vitamin

A daily, which resulted in a striking improvement in their tested driving efficiency. According to the Institute of Traffic Psychology in Karlsruhe, Germany, where the tests were conducted, after these dosages of vitamin A were given, more than half the drivers showed improvement in normal alertness lasting an average of six months.

Another German study in automobile driving shows that large amounts of vitamin C will sharpen those brain faculties that contribute to good and safe road behavior. Dr. A. Grossjohann, reporting in the journal *Arzneimittelforschung* (Pharmaceutical Research), stated that volunteers who had received large doses of vitamin C revealed a slight but clear increase of concentration power, understanding, coordination, and active response. People with those qualities are safe drivers, said Dr. Grossjohann. He advises that vitamin C should be taken before and during automobile trips.

Accident-Proneness

I would like to say a few words on the subject of accident-proneness. There are whole families that are accident prone. Some of them make comfortable livings from this tendency of theirs. They don't do it deliberately—they just can't help themselves. All kinds of theories are held for this, and psychiatrists and other medical men devote a lot of time to this problem. But I wonder how many of them have ever looked into the possibility that poor nutrition creates this kind of family. These people are usually of a lower grade—a sub-marginal group. Their minds are not nourished properly. They cannot make split-second decisions. They are easily confused. Many of these accident prone individuals drive cars.

Walter Dobson of Manchester University, England, recently said that we are living in "The Age of Inattention." We are developing a great mass of indifferent people who cannot concentrate on anything. This inattention, this drugged mental sense, this confused, fuzzy state of mind is national disease number one. It is the main contributor to accident-proneness, yet few doctors and experts have thought of national malnutrition as the basic cause of it. They overlook the progressive devitalization of our food, the increase in its chemicalization in the factories.

In a previous chapter I spoke of the energy-giving factors in desiccated liver. This supplement could be of tremendous value on long trips. Some drivers take dangerous drugs to be able to stay awake at the wheel for long periods. Desiccated liver not only furnishes extra energy, but gives an abundance of vitamin B which contributes to the health of the nervous system.

A recent research at Harvard, which comprised a survey of 11 northeastern states, revealed that auto drivers are "getting progressively more irritable in the squeeze of mounting traffic congestion." And it seems to be getting worse.

A weary truck driver told Harvard scientists how he was hurt in an accident when he saw a calf in the path of his moving truck. He swerved and overturned his vehicle. It was found later that there had been no calf there at all. It was just a "dream image," common to many persons who drive when they are too tired. If the truck driver had been a taker of desiccated liver tablets, this accident might have been prevented.

Sugary Sweets Not Advisable

Some drivers keep eating candy bars on long trips for energy. In fact, a few years ago I read a UPI news release to the effect that the National Safety Council is testing to see whether candy will keep drivers awake. The council said 60 Los Angeles truck drivers are being issued daily rations of chocolate bars, hard candies, and other confections. The drivers eat the sweets on the job and their reactions are recorded. . . . The release goes on to say that the rise in the blood sugar increases the alertness and performance ability. What the National Safety Council does not seem to know is that this candy eating practice will contribute to a *low* sugar state in the blood, and will lead to accident-prone possibilities. (See chapter on sugar.)

There have been dozens of medical studies of the motor accident problem reported in medical journals, and I have studied many of them, but nary a word will you find of the nutritional status of drivers as being a part of the cause. A typical one is an article by Geo. F. Strong, M.D., in *The Journal of the A.M.A.* of July 16, 1955. He suggests that the physical as well as psychiatric defects of automobile drivers be studied, but in "physical" he means diseases such as epilepsy, diabetes, alcoholism, and several others —but not one word on nutritional defects.

I have a news item before me, from the *New York Times* of July 27, 1957, which says that the Yale University Bureau of Highway Traffic admitted today that after 30 years of study it still did not know what caused automobile accidents. Professor Frederick W. Hurd, director of this Yale Bureau says, "No one has discovered the specific causes of accidents. We all know that speed and reckless driving kill thousands. But what makes one driver speed, and another reckless?" Professor Hurd doesn't have the slightest idea that it could be malnutrition. He has probably been brought up in the tradition that anyone who thinks in terms of malnutrition as a cause of disease is a food faddist.

The Human Factor

Dr. Stanley Mohler, director of the Civil Aeromedical Research Institute, in a recent speech at Oklahoma City (*Allentown Morning Call,* October 22, 1962), indicated the human factor as an important key to aviation safety. He said that man's reflexes, mental capabilities, and judgment have not improved while airplanes progressed from rattly 90-mile-an-hour biplanes to sleek jets that travel several times the speed of sound. He said the human factor —man's propensity to make errors—is closely linked with 9 out of 10 air accidents. Dr. Mohler's suggestions include a mild electrical shock which would cause mild pain but alert the pilot. This same effect could be produced through *super-nutrition.*

The same principles that apply to the automobile are also applicable to drivers of other vehicles—trains, planes, and ships. For example *The Philadelphia Inquirer* (April 2, 1962) says, "Multiple human errors rather than an act of God were blamed Sunday for the collapse of a radar tower which plunged 28 men to death in an Atlantic storm early last year." Many errors are caused by mental confusion of a brain not nourished properly.

An airplane disaster occurred some time ago in which it was discovered that someone at Zurich forgot to check the fuel on a Swiss Airliner going to London—a mere routine sort of thing. But when they were over the Channel and ran out of gas, 29 passengers drowned. Was it due to the fact that the gas-checker was addicted to Swiss chocolates, or smoked too much? Was his mind in a fog? This is an angle that the airlines should investigate.

A Remarkable Example

Before I close this chapter I would like to talk about John W. Jacobson, Director of the Accident Control Division of the F. J. Boutell Drive-Away Company of Flint, Michigan. This company has a fleet of those elongated trucks that transport automobiles. Mr. Jacobson became nutrition conscious from reading our *Prevention* magazine. He conducted an experiment which began in 1947, in which 18 drivers were chosen to whom a vitamin diet supplementation was made available at cost. The result? On the basis of a five year fleet average, these 18 men had a combined accident frequency of .28, or 357,143 miles per accident, as against .38 or 263,158 miles per accident for the rest of the company's drivers. This was a *35 percent reduction* for the 18 men who had supplemented their diet with vitamins.

There are people who are alive today and still walking around because of what these 18 men did, and it was done by nutrition.

In October, 1960, I addressed the Ohio and Pennsylvania Motor Truck Association Council of Safety Supervisors on the importance of diet in connection with motor truck accident prevention. This talk was printed, and a copy of it fell into the hands of H. K. Henderson, one of the truck drivers of the Boutell Company mentioned above. He became so enthusiastic about the possibility of accident reduction through vitamin taking that he obtained a distributorship for a line of natural, non-synthetic vitamin supplements, and decided upon an experiment.

He got 10 drivers of the Boutell Company to participate in a program of vitamin taking. The results after only one year were sensational. The experts will say it is impossible . . . but the facts are there. In the year before the experiment these 10 drivers had a total of two preventable vehicle accidents, four lost-time occupational injuries, and one injury with no loss of time. But in the year of the experiment, from July, 1961 to July, 1962, they rolled a total of 912,000 miles with not one vehicular accident, and not one occupational injury.

Henderson was chosen as one of a panel of eight, consisting of four outstanding drivers and four safety directors, at the Sheraton-Blackstone, on October 8th, 1962, their topic being, "How Can We Improve Our Safety Programs?" Henderson spoke mainly about the part that nutrition can play in accident prevention. He said, "Among other things that one of the drivers participating in the program is enjoying a complete reversal of personality. That is, from a notorious aggravator, non-conformist, militant individual to a most cooperative, enthusiastic employee. Some months ago, he was disagreeable, had a persecution complex, and as a union committee member was spending a great deal of his time rounding up grievances. If none were found, he would, reportedly, make every effort to foment some, at any and all opportunities. He was cited several times for discourtesy to customers. Yet, his performances and rampages were either of such a nature or just sufficiently infrequent that we were unable to effect a discharge.

"During the past several months he has been a one man public relations department for the company. He is very easy to get along with and at Committee meetings he is as docile as a dove, all smiles and speaks only when spoken to—or asked a question. He assists other drivers who may be having difficulties and berates those who appear to be careless or negligent. The transformation is something to behold!"

Add Vitamin A

In connection with what was shown by the German research with vitamin A, which indicated an improvement in the tested driving efficiency of 152 problem drivers, and also because of what I know about the ability of vitamin A in contributing to the body's quota of health, I am suggesting that we add vitamin A to our system, in the form of halibut liver oil perles. Thus, since halibut liver oil perles give us vitamin A and D, we are now taking vitamins A, B, C, D, and E.

I hope you are convinced that there is a relation between good diet and safe driving. For you it may spell additional years of healthy life, and less possibility of being crippled in an automobile accident. Standing alone, this chapter may not sound as convincing as if taken as part of the whole fabric. But as time goes on, and you see how much quicker your mind reacts at the wheel, you will be furnished with the most convincing proof—the proof of what it can do for *you*, aside from the proofs of medical researches and scientific principle.

15

Keeping the Thyroid Healthy

> *To have a brain that functions 100 percent, one's thyroid gland must be in a healthy state. This chapter will show you how certain persons become mentally ill due to the defective action of this gland.*
>
> *This is another reason why you must adopt all the suggestions contained in this book. They may help to correct any difficulties you may be having with your thyroid gland. But if something is radically wrong with it, see a doctor!*

HERE IS another case where, depending a great deal on nutrition, a physician did effective work with mental cases. I am talking about Nathan Masor, M.D., of Staten Island, N.Y. I read a paper he delivered to the Second International Congress for Psychiatry at Zurich, Switzerland (Sept. 1-7, 1957), in which he gave the details of 15 cases of mental disease with schizophrenic patterns which he had cured over a two-year period by means of thyroid hormones, vitamins, and a diet specific to each patient's problem, usually of high protein content. These cases were selected from hundreds who had also achieved favorable results. In this paper he advised the psychoanalysts to discard their couches.

Quoting from Dr. Masor's paper: "All patients treated . . . were acutely disturbed. They had been thoroughly processed in physical, X-ray, and laboratory examinations to insure that the conditions for which they were treated were solely psychiatric in nature. In every case there was a deterioration of personality, with element of affect (emotion) holding sway over the intellectual processes. Some had previously undergone shock therapy with equivocal results, but all had been subjected to prior psychiatric methods."

The medications used were a thyroid hormone, vitamin C, and vitamins of the B complex—namely, thiamine chloride, riboflavin, and niacinamide, which are known as oxytropic elements (whose net result is to improve the oxygen transport to the brain, via complex enzyme reactions). Another compound consisting of levo thyroxin, which is the hormone of the thyroid gland, and Vitamin B_{12}, by injection, were the other medicaments used.

Three Cases

The following are descriptions of three of the cases given in Dr. Masor's paper, abbreviated in detail because of limitation on speaking time at the Congress Hall.

M.D., married, age 47, a woman whose tenseness is reflected in anxious fancies, rapid speech, and tremulousness. Chief complaint over many years' standing was "nervous stomach." There was difficulty in concentration and she became very unsocial. Gastro-intestinal X-ray series and other tests were negative. Multiplicity of other complaints, from chest pains to vertigo were present. She had previously been given a great deal of sedatives, different physicians, and a series of fourteen shock treatments, with no lasting beneficial effects. She could not finish a day's work due to exhaustion. Insomnia was another prominent complaint. It took only five weekly injections of the thyroid hormone and B_{12} and the oral medication, starting March 1957, to effectuate a virtual reversal of above symptoms. There had been a complete eradication of the stomach complaints, exhaustive state and side complaints, and she states that she has never felt as emotionally secure as within the five weeks of treatment, with improvement starting after the third week.

F.M., widow, 51. With the onset of her menopausal state, a change in personality from a social, pleasant woman to a withdrawn, depressed one occurred. Besides lack of energy, palpitation, insomnia, etc., she would perform numerous useless movements with her hands. Her favorite preoccupation during these frequent sieges was to constantly tear paper into pieces. It was six weeks before there was any evidence of improvement with oxytropic factors. Her emotional state continued progressively well, except for some transient setbacks which were eliminated by an increase in dosage to slightly higher levels. She has since remained satisfactorily symptom-free, with interval treatments of two to four weeks.

W.A., a 48-year-old single woman, complaining of constipation, exhaustion, tremulousness, insomnia. Weight 87½ pounds at start of treatment, on January 27, 1957. Was unable to raise arms. She felt as tired on arising as on going to bed. Shunned people. She became increasingly irritable and developed delusions of reference with her associates. She was placed on therapy, with oxytropic factors, and received weekly injection to April 20th (except for one week). On high caloric intake and therapy, her most recent weight was 101½ pounds. Her constipation began to go away. She felt much calmer. She sleeps through the night and feels refreshed, even if she sleeps only five or six hours. Her stamina, ambition, and social attitudes are markedly improved.

Psychiatry, a Backward Procedure

Dr. Masor believes that psychiatry may be attacking the problem backwards in delving into past emotional events rather than considering them as offspring of the disease, so to speak. He says,

> Few patients gain stability by probing the half-forgotten past. It is fortunate for all of us that the healthy mind suppresses the objectionable experiences and recalls with ease the pleasurable moments previously spent; else, relaxation and peace of mind would not be possible. Why then should the mentally ill be subjected to the scrutiny of his unconsciousness when his balance to start with is much more delicate than that of the normal person? The purposeful elevation of such well-repressed impressions to cortical (outward) cognizance often only leads to a compounding and prolonging of his painful impressions. May not, as a consequence, such a procedure lead to an aggravation of the mental state rather than amelioration? Might it not be well for the psychiatrist to try to effectuate the reverse by attempting to drive the patient's ever-present cortical neurotic and painful impressions to the deeper subthalmic level?

The biochemical (dietetic) approach described

here seems to be a more fundamental treatment for nervous ailments than any provided by a purely psychiatric approach. Moreover, its simplicity, directness and economy give it distinct advantages. While it is the basic step, we should keep in mind that the biochemical method is only the first step and that it must be followed up in almost every case by psychological or psychiatric work which would have the main function of aiding in the re-education of the patient and assisting him in adapting adequately to his newly acquired mental and physical status.

A Healthy Thyroid Gland Important

A well-functioning thyroid is necessary because the secretions from this gland help the oxygen to be transported through the body. Drs. Danziger and Kindwall (*Diseases of the Nervous System*, August, 1948) stated that all mental disorders are symptoms of *anoxia* (oxygen deficiency), and in working with a series of 19 psychotic (insane) patients, they cured the deficiency by feeding them large doses of thyroid extract, and thus cleared up the psychosis.

They could have speeded up results if they had given their patients vitamins B and E, which are associated in maintaining the oxygenation of the body.

So, if you want to stay mentally healthy, look to the health of your thyroid. Of course, there are other causes of mental disease, but the under-active thyroid is a prominent one.

Now, how do we *maintain* a healthy thyroid? I think the first rule is to be generally healthy—a sound thyroid in a sound body! We must, therefore, be health conscious. Secondly, we must be sure of our iodine supply. All sea foods are rich in iodine. There are limited amounts in eggs, meats, vegetables, nuts, etc., but the best source is in kelp tablets. Two or three kelp tablets a day and you can forget about your iodine needs.

Anti-Thyroid Factors

Shall we take iodized salt? In *Endocrinology* (56:387, 1955), mice tested for goiter-activating foods showed that an enlargement of the thyroid could be caused by salt. With the omission of salt, the goiters went back to their normal size.

Aspirin has an immediate anti-thyroid action, says *The Journal of Endocrinology* (Nov. 1953), and low thyroid action is often the result of its use. In other words, the taking of aspirin by some people could cause mental symptoms.

In *The Journal of the A.M.A.* (Nov. 23, 1957), Dr. Arnold S. Jackson wrote that "the most important single factor responsible for symptoms of thyroid disturbance in 228 patients he observed was the over-indulgence in the use of stimulants—coffee, tea, and nicotine." Many of these patients smoked two or three packs of cigarettes a day, and drank from five to thirty cups of coffee each day!

Kathy

There is a story about a girl called "Kathy" which is described in a book by that name, published in 1957 by E. P. Dutton Company. Kathy was a young girl who changed with alarming rapidity from a normal healthy child to a shadow. Her weight steadily dropped. Her good spirits and energy simply disappeared and she suffered from a frustrating inability to keep warm. One doctor after another was consulted, and each was forced to admit that he could find nothing wrong with Kathy. As a last resort, the child was taken to a psychiatrist who declared that she was suffering from a psychosis and should be sent to a mental hospital.

Almost by accident, shortly thereafter, she happened to be in the office of an M.D. who decided to test the operation of her thyroid gland. He found it dangerously deficient, and gave her a thyroxin preparation to supplement the short supply in her body. In a matter of hours, her condition was noticeably improved. In a few weeks her terrible ordeal was over and she was back at school, a perfectly normal girl. Without the alertness of this M.D., Kathy might have been condemned to years of confinement in a mental institution and, eventually, to a premature death.

Cronin's Novel

About 25 years ago or more, doctor-novelist A. J. Cronin, in his book *Between Two Worlds*, described a classic case of a patient with an underactive thyroid, whose physician recommended his admittance to a mental institution, without thinking that a thyroid disorder could be the cause. Cronin repeated the description again in one of his most famous novels, *The Citadel.* He describes the symptoms of hypothyroidism as including defective memory, slow mentation, and attacks of irritability, culminating in an outburst of homicidal violence. Reading that makes one wonder how many of the beds in our mental hospitals are taken by patients who need nothing more than additional thyroxin in their diet to become as mentally normal as any of us.

In a *Reader's Digest* article (February, 1959), science writer Albert Maisel writes of a survey which shows that 8½ million Americans are victims of hypothyroidism (low thyroid action), and we presume that very few of these are aware of it. A slowing thyroid may not be suspected, even when its function is 15 to 20 percent below normal. At this stage, the victim has vague and chronic symptoms such as fatigue, muscle weakness, headaches, constipation, nasal congestion, menstrual disturbance, or just a general feeling of being below par. A difficulty of diagnosis in thyroid cases is that anxiety over some problem may so elevate the reading that it might falsely indicate a normal thyroid function.

The relation between subnormal thyroid activity and mental health has been noted in medical writings. *The British Medical Journal* (May 26, 1951) told of testing 541 psycho-neurotic and psychotic patients. Over 50 percent of the males showed a tendency toward below-normal thyroid function. In *Postgraduate Medicine* (9:400 in 1951), a Dr. Layey made the amazing statement: "We have always known that hypothyroidism is related to the emotional states."

In *The Canadian Medical Association Journal* (Dec. 15, 1956), Drs. Ferguson and Rayport noted that the thyroid is known to have a direct connection with the central nervous system of the body. In a news release from the Lehigh County (Pa.) Medical Society, in the *Allentown Morning Call* (Jan. 2, 1958), it is stated that an emotionally distraught person may go to a psychiatrist, thinking he has mental trouble, when his real problem is an underactive thyroid gland. And, in the *New York Times* of Nov. 8, 1959 it was stated that at Cornell, based on researches extending over three years, it was reported that certain patients with serious mental illnesses are abnormal in the way their bodies use thyroid hormones. So, we are pretty sure of our ground when we say that, given a healthy thyroid, there is less chance of becoming mentally ill than where there is a deranged thyroid metabolism.

REVIEW

We at *Prevention* maintain that if our entire system is practiced, all the organs of the body, including the thyroid gland, will be helped. If, however, one has the symptoms described in this chapter it might be well to have one's thyroid checked by a physician. But be sure to add kelp tablets to your daily vitamin program. You will be taking a lot of tablets. I take over 60 a day, but they are all food products, not synthetic high-powered drugs. It takes work at first, but you will soon get into the habit, and it will eventually become second nature.

16

Getting Youngsters Started Right

Are you a juvenile delinquent? Then this chapter is for you. Are you an adult delinquent? Then read this chapter twice. Probably we all have some criminal tendencies in our make-up, but by improving our general health, as will surely occur if one follows the entire system described in this book, that tendency could be reduced to the vanishing point!

The situation is becoming very dangerous. Crime seems to be increasing too much each year. What can you do to help the situation after you have read this chapter?

ONE ASSURING thought you will get from reading this chapter is that you might cure yourself of any criminal tendencies lying dormant under the surface. This book gives an impression that the diet can improve the mentality. But, as Dr. Berman has been quoted as saying (Chapter 7), it can also improve one's character, even to making you a model citizen.

The people concerned with the crime problem, especially that of juvenile deliquency, do not seem to be aware that food has anything to do with it. They scoff at such suggestions. While they do, the crime rate seems to be going up and up, until one of these days it won't be safe for anyone to walk down any side street at night, or perhaps even in the daytime.

All kinds of reasons are presented for the juvenile delinquency problem, but the main one seems to be that these hoodlums come from broken homes. Well I have news for them. This is not so. In the "Midtown Community Health Study" of Manhattan, N.Y. (*Public Health Reports,* November, '63), appears the following: "Almost all the social ills to which man is heir have been laid at the door of the broken home, including juvenile delinquency, drug addiction, and mental disease." The data gathered seemed to show that this is true only under certain rare conditions. In the conclusion of the article there is the statement, "We have found that broken homes are not strongly associated with mental disorder."

A Startling Survey

I will tell you something more significant about certain homes, which are not exactly "broken up." In a survey made a few years ago of 3,000 juvenile delinquents in New York City, it was found that on the average they had only three meals a week at home—three meals out of a possible 21. The rest of the time they were no doubt consuming a typical jitterbug diet in candy stores and cheap luncheonettes. It is my considered opinion that we can feed our young ones into decency, and even honesty.

A most interesting example of the effect of a healthy diet on character appeared in the *London Sunday Chronicle* of May 3, 1953, under the heading, "Diet Makes Naughty Girls Good." It follows:

> Can diet cut juvenile delinquency?
>
> A just-completed survey of 17 maladjusted or delinquent girls between the ages of 11 and 15 in a Camberwell (London) Salvation Army hostel seems to prove it can.
>
> Previously the girls lived on the poorest possible type of meal: white bread and margarine, cheap jam, lots of sweet tea, tinned and processed meats.
>
> Fish and chips had been one of their most nutritious meals.
>
> But a year ago in Springfield Lodge their diet was changed to raw fruit, nuts, vegetables, salads, wholewheat bread, dates, prunes, figs, honey,

cheese, meat, fish, eggs, crushed wheat, and oatmeal.

And this is what happened:

They quickly became less aggressive and less quarrelsome, bad habits seemed to disappear, "problem children" became less of a problem, and the bored ones lost their boredom.

Physically, they improved almost beyond recognition.

Major Hudson, the warden, told me last night: "It is amazing to see the difference in their complexions, general brightness, and poise. But the difference in their behavior is the most significant.

"The part the diet has played in their personalities is undeniable."

Institutional Malnutrition

In an investigation in New York (*New York State Journal of Medicine*, 1954, Vol. 45, page 74), it was found that there were evidences of malnutrition in not less than 80 percent of 750 boys admitted to an institution for juvenile delinquents.

Denver Juvenile Court Judge Philip B. Gillian recently said that a major cause of juvenile delinquency is an improper diet; it generally was the root of school maladjustments, decreased alertness, and lowered efficiency. He suggested better knowledge of nutrition on the part of the parents.

Ezra T. Benson, former Secretary of the U.S. Department of Agriculture, told a Lincoln Day dinner audience at the National Youthpower Congress that there are great deficiencies in the diet of teenagers. Regarding this talk, the *New York Times* (Feb. 18, 1960) quoted him: "Lack of knowledge about proper eating was a factor in the weakening of American family life and the rise of juvenile delinquency."

In the *New York Times* (March 27, 1960), in an article "Youths Suffering from Poor Diets," appears the following: "School work and alertness suffer when the teenage body is lacking in vital food elements. It shows up in bad temper, acne, or loss of stamina. . . . The long term results are impaired health and a weakening of future generations. Malnutrition is sometimes connected with juvenile delinquency."

The "Beatster"

Here is an excerpt from a letter sent by Harold N. Simpson, a biochemist, to *The National Review* (May 23, 1959). It is in reference to Ernest Van den Haag's discussion of the "beat" generation in the April 11 issue. Simpson says:

"You look into the diet of these 'beatsters.' Believe me, you raise a child on buns and hamburgers, white bread and hot dogs, ice cream and cokes, and you end up with a juvenile delinquent on your hands. When the quality of the diet declines, the person is not able to think straight."

Myril Axelrod, writing in *The Reader's Digest* (December 1955), made a tour of high school cafeterias. He found well-balanced meals ignored in favor of hot dogs and soft drinks. In one place, out of 1500 students, only 90 ate in the school dining room where they could eat a balanced meal. The rest ate at snack bars and hot dog wagons.

He said, "I stood on the balcony of a large cafeteria opposite a boys' high school and watched the trays go by. While the counters displayed soups, meats, salads, vegetables, and fruits, the students' trays bore, instead, macaroni, baked beans, bread, cake, pies, ice cream, and coffee."

Pennsylvania State College studied the food habits of 2,536 teen-agers and found that only about a quarter of them were eating according to the recommendations of the National Research Council for Good Nutrition.

Psychiatry Ignores Nutrition

The psychiatrists seem to ignore the dining room as a factor in the cause of juvenile delinquency. They continue operating in their rut, writing articles which only tend to confuse the issues. John Crosby said in the *New York Herald Tribune* (May 21, 1962), "The experts in juvenile delinquency are getting to be voodoo priests talking their own mumbo jumbo that doesn't seem to be meaning anything or apply to anything."

Their idea to solve juvenile delinquency is to put more cops on the beat, build more institutions to house them, appropriate more Congressional money, pass laws to make it a crime for a youth to carry a knife, mobilize youth for various purposes, arrest parents of delinquents and put *them* in jail, treat delinquents with kid gloves, use force on them, whip them if necessary, use every possible resource (I am reading these from newspaper clippings I have collected), issue warnings, establish a good emotional climate to provide a vicarious outlet for their aggressive feelings, improve the more traditional correctional services of probation, parole, and institutional facilities, create a major national blueprint, give delinquent youngsters skating and music lessons, and trips to Greenwich Village coffee houses, get girl scouts to help, turn the problem over to family doctors, attack the problem "across the board," organize urban young service corps, etc., but practically never a word about improved nutrition for youth.

Suggestion

The suggestion that comes nearest to the best solution is to create work camps on farms for these delinquents. I am all for these, provided the boys and girls raise their own food there, eat a wholesome nutritious diet, and are taught the facts of nutrition, so that when they go back home they can continue to maintain their mental health by consuming a healthy diet.

Now let us go a little more in detail into the effect of diet on juvenile delinquency. E. E. Dudding, of the Prisoner's Relief Society, wrote a letter to the *Washington* (D.C.) *Daily News* which was published in its Feb. 2, 1960 issue as follows:

> We have found in returning convicts, a high percentage of the men released from the nation's prisons are afflicted with chronic acidosis; that is, the blood is too acid. In the early days of the Prisoner's Relief Society we discovered nearly all the inmates of our prisons were suffering with acidosis when they entered, and were still afflicted when released. We traced it to the prison food. Acidosis affects the mind to such an extent that a man is hardly able to take care of himself.
>
> After much research we developed a short cure for acidosis and practiced it for 40 years. But we found it was a law violation to prescribe the diet we used. The District Board of Medical Examiners ordered us to stop. I think this explains the crime epidemic in Washington.

Foods that are very acid and that contribute to acidosis are sugar, bread, cereals, cakes, etc.

Very valuable work in the field of low blood sugar was done by Joseph Wilder, M.D. of New York City. In the April (1943-1944) issue of *The Nervous Child*, Dr. Wilder published the results of work which proved conclusively that there is a direct connection between a person's low blood sugar and the tendency to be a criminal. In some cases it merely turns people into neurotics; it makes others "difficult." Bear in mind that low blood sugar usually comes from a high consumption of sugar, as explained in Chapter 2.

Low Blood Sugar Symptoms

Here are some of the symptoms Dr. Wilder has found in patients suffering from low blood sugar: slowing of mental processes, dullness, difficulty in making even minor decisions, depression, anxiety, irritability, and tendency to be negative; also physical symptoms like double vision, dizziness, changes in voice texture, and so forth.

Some of the symptoms of low blood sugar in children are overeating or not wanting to eat at all. Impairment of memory in the form of amnesia is one of the most common happenings in more severe cases of low blood sugar. When the child states that he did not do or say a certain thing, he may actually not remember. The child may not sleep well. Nightmares, sleep-walking, or even bed-wetting may be symptoms. He does not learn. "The child may be neurotic, psychopathic, or have criminal tendencies," says Dr. Wilder. "And be subject to anxiety, running away tendencies, aggressiveness, a blind urge to activity, and destructiveness with impairment of moral sensibilities like shame. In its simplest form, it is the tendency to deny everything, contradict everything, refuse everything at any price. . . . It is no wonder that a considerable number of criminal and semi-criminal acts have been observed in children in *hypoglycemic* (low blood sugar) states, ranging from destructiveness or violation of traffic regulations, all the way to bestiality, arson, and homicide."

Strong statements indeed, to be based on the observations of one person only! But Dr. Wilder's beliefs were tested in Argentina by researchers N. Rojas and A. F. Sanchi, who wrote an article on "Hypoglycemia and Delinquents" which appeared in the *Archives of Legal Medicine*, volume 11, page 29, 1941. In this article they told of doing blood sugar tests on a group of apprehended delinquents. There was a striking percentage with low, sometimes *extremely* low, blood sugar.

In an article which appeared in the *Handbook of Correctional Psychology*, published in 1947, Dr. Wilder says,

"Criminal acts have been committed time and again in abnormal psychological conditions impairing judgment or self-control." In this article Dr. Wilder proceeds to discuss many well-documented cases of criminal acts performed by individuals suffering from low blood sugar. Tests indicated, without a shadow of a doubt, that each individual was in a state of low blood sugar at the time the crime was committed. The crimes range all the way from homicide to sadism, arson, serious traffic violations, mutilation, violent aggressiveness, etc. In fact, the article sounds as if you might be reading today's and yesterday's newspaper.

WHAT TO DO

With all this medical evidence of the relation of malnutrition to criminal tendencies, is it not strange that, in the usual meetings of the authorities to discuss and study the question of delinquency, not a word is said about nutrition? In the last few weeks of writing this book, several Columbia University professors have been attacked by juvenile delinquents. Should not then the professional world concern itself more with this rising problem which is becoming more acute each year, especially since it is hitting home?

They read about these happenings, shake their heads, and think that the psychiatrists are doing all they can to come up with a solution. It is a world of specialization. If the problem were properly considered, perhaps a mathematics or a chemistry or a biology professor might be more apt to find the answer. They all should get into the act, and *soon,* or there is nothing to expect but a hopeless chaos. The present system will never dig out the truth from the mess of psychiatric gibberish that emerges from each juvenile delinquency conclave.

The juvenile delinquent is suffering from a "sugar confusion." He cannot think straight. He does not know why he is breaking the law. The answer may be as simple as to place police in the candy stores to prevent sugar products from being sold to minors, just as they do with liquor. Perhaps social workers should be placed in these stores, first to convince these store-keepers to have fruit and other healthy food for sale, and secondly to teach the young rowdy element that their lives would be happier if they passed up the soft drinks, ice-creams, and candies.

And the same to you, dear reader. In your desk at work, hide some fruit rather than the usual candy bars. You will gain by feeling an increase of mental energy, a greater clarity of thinking ability, a general increase in mental power, and less cavities.

17

The Prevention
Magazine Program

> *In this chapter we make suggestions for further improvement in your diet, albeit with no direct evidence with regard to their effect on the action of the mind. But we do know that their adoption by you will be effective in improving your general health. And since the general health contributes so much to brain health, you will certainly want to read this chapter carefully and see how you can work the ideas contained therein into your new program of diet.*

As YOU MAY already know, the writer is the editor of *Prevention*, the largest independent health magazine in the world. But *Prevention* is really not a magazine—it is a system. You have already been given much of this system, but there are still other things that you can do which can contribute to creating optimum health.

Our theme is simple. The healthier you are, the better your mind will be able to function, provided you also give it some mental gymnastics to do. So, if you want to get the maximum abilities out of your mind, go the whole way. Take it all! But you don't have to do it all at one gulp. Here are a few ideas for your eventual adoption.

Bread

Bread has no place in the *Prevention* system. It is not the staff of life, even though it is whole wheat. Bread is fattening, constipating, ferments in the stomach, causes heart symptoms in many heart patients and celiac disease in children (a disease which distends the abdomen). It also brings on diarrhea and other disagreeable symptoms —this is quite common in children. If all wheat products are cut from the diet, sensational cures are obtained. If there is not sufficient vitamin D in the diet, eating wheat and wheat cereals will cause rickets. It is also a factor in bringing on colds. It is a highly acid food, and takes extremely long to be digested, causing a state of lowered body defenses against the cold germ or virus. It causes many other disease conditions too numerous to mention here. Try a breadless and grainless diet for a month and see what it will do for you. This means cutting out bread, cereals, cakes, spaghetti, noodles, gravy, etc. By cutting out this form of starch you will have to fill up on more vegetables and protein. We do favor the wheat germ of the wheat as well as the bran, for it is the starch portion, including the gluten, that does the harm. To me this proscription against bread is one of the most important planks in the *Prevention* system, and applies to the organically-raised wheat as well as that raised with chemical fertilizers.

Citrus Fruits

In past issues of *Prevention,* we have presented evidence from medical and dental journals indicating that large quantities of citrus fruit juices may harm teeth and health in general. Individuals who are especially sensitive have found that by omitting citrus juice they have cleared up stubborn cases of bleeding gums, headaches, and fatigue. We suggest that citrus fruits be eaten—not juiced—and eaten in extreme moderation. Drinking orange juice has caused extremely painful cases of itching rectum. This goes for oranges, grapefruit, and lemons. Our attitude is based on medical research. To be on the safe side, eat no citrus at all. Otherwise, do so only in extreme moderation!

Milk

We are not in favor of adults drinking milk—and for children, it should only be used in moderation. Dairy food has been found to be a factor in making children grow tall. There is medical evidence that very tall people are not as healthy as shorter ones. They have more high blood pressure, back and foot troubles, and don't live as long. But tall folks need not worry if they follow the *Prevention* system. It will counteract the effect of the tallness.

Modern milk, based on the artificial practices of agriculture and because of its pasteurization, is a far cry from old-fashioned raw milk. Its growth factor, which is supposed to help children, may be dangerous for adults. Excellent health can be maintained without milk. Take bonemeal tablets instead.

There are many conditions and allergies that come from milk drinking. It is too complicated a subject to cover here, but—no milk, butter, cheese, ice-cream, etc. A trial will convince you.

Olive Oil

We are strongly in favor of olive oil. It is wonderful for ulcer sufferers. It can harden the gums, and of late, in Spain, research has been done to show that it is a protection against radiation. Take a spoonful before each meal.

Unsaturated Fatty Acids

These are essential from a nutrition standpoint, because the body cannot manufacture them. They occur in unprocessed natural fats chiefly of vegetable origin, such as cereal and vegetable oils like salad oils, olive oil, corn oil, and peanut oil; also in avocadoes, nuts, and, of course, sunflower seeds and other seeds. These are the fatty substances which prevent cholesterol deposits in the blood vessels.

Animal fats contain little of these important fatty acids, and this is one reason why it is believed that a diet high in animal fats and low in vegetable fats causes cholesterol deposits. When vegetable fats are hydrogenated (that is, made solid), they are changed chemically and the essential fatty acids are largely destroyed.

We advise keeping to a minimum the animal fat in the diet and shunning hydrogenated fats (solid ones like margarine and the canned shortenings). Salad oils and other sources of vegetable fats are good for you.

The whole subject of the effect of cholesterol on the body is full of conflict and controversy. It probably is safest to cut out fats such as those from milk, butter, lard, etc. But include oils such as safflower, corn, soybean, sunflower seed, olive, etc. Safflower is supposed to be best for reducing cholesterol in the blood.

Lecithin—a fatty substance occurring with cholesterol in foods. It is believed that lecithin renders the cholesterol harmless. Anyone fearing hardening of the arteries or high blood pressure should get plenty of lecithin. You get it in natural foods, not in refined foods. Eggs and unprocessed vegetable oils are rich sources of lecithin. You can also get it in capsule form at health food stores. We recommend a capsule at each meal.

Rutin—a substance that occurs with vitamin C in foods. It is used in concentrated form as a treatment for high blood pressure and to strengthen the walls of the blood vessels. It can be obtained in health food stores.

Bone Meal—Lack of calcium, magnesium, phosphorus, and other minerals is one of our most serious diet deficiencies, resulting in tooth decay and scores of other ailments. Bone meal provides them in completely natural form. Take bone meal every day—either in tablet or powdered form.

Bone meal prevents tooth cavities, strengthens the bones against fracture, and has a beneficial effect on the pulse and heart.

Water (Drinking)—If you do not have your own well or spring, it is best to drink purchased spring water, for it does not contain added chlorine or other chemicals. Chlorine uses up vitamin E in the body. As a rule also aluminum sulphate is used in public drinking water. No research has ever been done on the long-term effects of drinking chlorinated water.

Water-Softeners—If you use a water-softener, have it work on the hot water faucet only. To drink artificially softened water is extremely dangerous. The water softening process produces a chemical action in which calcium and magnesium are removed and sodium is placed into the water. This is the equivalent of adding salt to the water. Calcium and magnesium are both of tremendous value to good health.

Utensils (Aluminum)

Never use aluminum cooking utensils. Aluminum is a soft, toxic metal and some of it will get into the hot water of the cooked mineral and contaminate it. It causes digestive troubles in some people, and will usually raise the pulse. Pyrex glass, enamelware, and stainless steel are better, in the order mentioned. There is a huge amount of evidence that cooking in aluminum utensils is dangerous.

Utensils (Plastic)

Plastic utensils should never be used for food or drink. They contain harmful chemical poisons, like formaldehyde, which may get into the food. It is difficult to sterilize them, and even in hospitals water in such containers has been found to contain harmful bacteria.

So, our system entails not only adding vitamins, but also watching the diet carefully to eliminate certain foods and to add others. This will not be accomplished in a week. Do it gradually, item by item, and watch the interesting effects not only on your mind, but on your health generally.

18

Natural vs. Synthetic Vitamins

Here is a new concept in connection with the taking of vitamins, probably one you have never heard of—that there is a difference between vitamin B and vitamin B. The vitamins that you get in your drug store are probably of the synthetic, coal-tar variety.

I feel that it is best to take vitamins that are extracted from foods, rather than being built up from chemical building blocks, and in this chapter you will be given medical evidence to show why the natural ones are better for you.

CLARENCE BUDINGTON KELLAND in one of his stories had a character remark, "Leave our chemists alone and they'll be able to give you synthetic strawberries." Well, many people who are taking vitamins today are getting the equivalent of synthetic strawberries—compounds made usually from coal tar. There's a whale of a difference between a synthetic and a natural product.

I will give you an example. Many people today do not exercise. As a result their adrenal glands don't make enough cortisone, and, for lack of it, many may come down with arthritis. Then they are given artificially made cortisone in which there are many gaps. No pharmaceutical chemist can make cortisone like the adrenals can. The result is that serious side-effects result from the taking of this man-made cortisone—side effects such as the weakening of the spine and brain.

Two biochemists working in the laboratories of Distillation Products Industries, the pharmaceutical division of

Eastman Kodak, spent two years comparing the natural with the synthetic vitamin E. The two products were seemingly identical in composition, but they found that the I-somer in the synthetic vitamin E had only 20.6 per cent as much biological activity as the I-somer in the natural vitamin E. In other words, though they seem to be chemical twins, the natural vitamin E is five times as active and five times as effective as the synthetic.

Incidentally, if you wish to know what an I-somer is, it is a substance that has the same composition, in different variations of it, but has different chemical or physical properties.

The poisonous nature of the synthetic vitamin D sold as *Viosterol* and *Vigantol* is well established. It causes blood to form in the urine of children very quickly, by its destructive action to the kidneys. Deaths have been reported from the ordinary dosages used to "protect" from rickets. (*Journal of the American Medical Association* 130:1208-1215, 1946.) We get natural vitamin A plus vitamin D in halibut liver oil perles.

Niacin is another of the B complex vitamins that can be made only in the synthetic form. It is often used in ground meat, to "assure retention of its color," says *Consumer's Bulletin* (March, 1962). "In Philadelphia, Pennsylvania, two cases of niacin poisoning involving five persons were reported in 1961 that involved the same symptoms, intense flushing of the skin, a feeling of warmth, itching, and some abdominal discomfort." In the natural method, a person gets his niacin and pantothenic acid from brewer's yeast, wheat germ, and desiccated liver, with no harmful effects.

In the same way when nicotinic acid was added to ground meat to prevent darkening of the meat, outbreaks of food poisoning occurred. This happened to 88 persons out of 145 as described in *The Nebraska Medical Journal* 42:243-245, May, 1957. Nicotinic acid is another fraction of the B complex which is obtainable in a natural form from brewer's yeast, etc. In the case just mentioned, it was produced synthetically.

The Journal of the American Medical Association (May 3, 1952) describes a severe shock with collapse in a 57-year-old physician who received thiamine injections. Several other cases of thiamine intolerances are described in *Annals of Allergy*, May 1952, pages 291 to 307. This never happens to people getting thiamine from whole natural products like brewer's yeast, wheat germ, or desiccated liver.

A clinical experience is related in the *Canadian Medical Association Journal* (volume 44, page 20, 1941). Fifteen cases of skin disease were treated with injections of synthetic vitamin B. There was no improvement noted from these treatments until yeast or liver extract was given. Observing physicians noted that a general beneficial effect was then obtained.

Take the case of vitamin C. The natural product can be taken in the form of products made from rose hips, red peppers, or the acerola cherry, and it can be made synthetically in the form of pure ascorbic acid. The difference is that the natural product is not pure. However, its so-called impurities are in the form of other vitamins and minerals. This is highly desirable from a curative viewpoint. A balanced package is superior to a narrow, purified fragment.

Let me cite an experiment which was performed behind the Iron Curtain, and which was reported in the Russian medical journal called *Vitamin Research News*, No. 1, 40 (1946). Mice were fed a deficient diet which is known to produce scurvy, and when it was apparent that they were all suffering from this disease they were divided into two groups and treated with vitamin C, which is known to cure this condition. But one group was given the vitamin produced synthetically while the other had the benefit of vitamin C obtained from a plant. The group that was fed on the natural vitamin C was completely cured within a short time, but not the other.

A book published in 1936, by the U.S. Vitamin Co., called *Vitamin and Mineral Therapy*, by E. H. Dubin and Casimir Funk (the latter the man who discovered vitamin B), contains the following statement, "Synthetic vitamins: These are highly inferior to vitamins from natural sources, also, the synthetic product is well known to be far more toxic."

The American Review of Tuberculosis, volume 72, page 218, 1955, describes a study of failures of vitamin A metabolism in TB patients. Synthetic vitamin A and cod liver oil were given. "The response was much better with the cod liver oil concentrate than with synthetic vitamin A," say the authors.

In spite of this difference between natural and the synthetic, the *Journal of the American Medical Association* says, as quoted in *Cosmopolitan* (December 21, 1940), "There is no detectable difference between the synthetic chemical vitamin and the natural ones. Ascorbic acid is just as good vitamin C as one gets from an orange." This was in 1940. In 1958 (December 13) the *Journal of the American Medical Association* said the same thing, namely, "Whether the body obtains its vitamin C from synthetic ascorbic acid or from orange juice, the manner in which this substance is utilized by the body is exactly the same."

But Dr. Alexander Berglas, a physician connected with the Pasteur Institute, said, "In spite of the therapeutic value of synthetic vitamins in the treatment of certain diseases, one should not believe that the mere ingestion of the pure synthetic vitamins, even if identical in chemical structure to the natural vitamins, necessarily has the same effect on our body as the consumption of vitamins in combination with their natural concomitants. The latter are not to be dismissed as 'excess baggage,' but must be thought of as the result of millions of years of evolution of optimal combinations."

A remarkable experiment was done jointly at the University of Southern California and the University of California at Los Angeles, supervised by Drs. George Watson and Andrew L. Comrey, and written up in *The Journal of Psychology* (1954, 38, pp. 251-264). They treated a test group of 32 emotionally disturbed persons with pills containing vitamins and minerals. Twenty-nine of them improved, 15 of them markedly. In a control group of 11 persons who were given placebo pills (sugar filled), only one improved.

The doctors had a drug company make pills for them containing practically every known vitamin and mineral, plus other food supplements. The interesting thing is the number of natural substances in this formula, as well as items that are in the *Prevention* system. These include vitamin A and D (Halibut liver oil), vitamin E, soya lecithin, wheat germ, kelp, bone meal, red bone marrow, liver, alfalfa, parsley, escarole, watercress, etc.

Says the *Syracuse Herald* (Oct. 27, 1954) regarding this experiment, "Joseph M. Stanton, district supervisor of the California State Vocational Rehabilitation Department . . . said, 'The implications are enormous. This new therapy could be of great help and simplification in treating some types of mental illness.' "

Stanton said that a similar experiment had been carried

out at a private sanitarium for the mentally ill in Los
Angeles.

There, he said, a control was run on patients who were
given the vitamin therapy or electric shock treatment. He
said results indicated strongly that the nutritional therapy
was more helpful in every case studied than the more
drastic and sometimes potentially dangerous shock system.

In 1955 I wrote a little book of 64 pages called *Is Our
Intelligence Declining?* (Rodale Press), in which some of
the researches mentioned here were included. I sent the
proofs of it to Dr. Andrew L. Comrey, Watson's associate
in the experiments just described, and the following is a
letter he wrote to me:

> Feb. 14, 1955
>
> Mr. J. I. Rodale
> Allentown, Pa.
> Dear Sir:
>
> Thank you for allowing me to read the proof
> of your book *Is Our Intelligence Declining?* I
> find what you have to say well supported and
> reasonable. Whether people who *should* will pay
> any attention to it is something else again. There
> seems to be an unofficial but highly organized
> conspiracy among the majority to regard propon-
> ents of good nutrition as public nuisances if not
> dangerous quacks attempting to practice medi-
> cine without a license. I wish you success in your
> crusade. I shall, and am doing what I can to
> support it.
>
> I sent your original letter to Dr. Watson. He
> will no doubt send you a reprint of our original
> article on this topic which adds evidence to sup-
> port your statements.
>
> Thank you very much for your interest. I am
> returning your proof under separate cover.
>
> Cordially,
> Andrew L. Comrey
> Assistant Professor

There are big interests selling huge amounts of synthetic
vitamins and other substances, and they are in the driver's
seat in regard to teaching the public what is right and what
is wrong about vitamins. They call us food faddists without
proving that we are wrong. We seem to be food faddists

because we are different. Yes, we *are* different—the results you get from natural products are so different!

The average doctor is so used to prescribing drugs that it is not foreign to his philosophy to prescribe synthetic vitamins, which are in the same category as drugs. But in the natural food concept, we question the effect of such synthetics after 20 or 30 years of usage. In many drugs the dangerous side-effects show themselves at once, but in the milder synthetic, coal tar vitamins, these effects may be slower in coming, but they might come later, and *I* don't want to be made a guinea pig. In our type of natural food supplement vitamins, there cannot possibly be any dangerous side-effects, now or later.

19

Kick Drugs Out of Your Life

> *If you are a regular taker of aspirins, or if you have been given drugs by your doctor more or less regularly, you are creating a condition of fogginess in your mental work. These drugs are usually highly soluble and rush into the bloodstream, and there create imbalances. Many of them destroy vitamins.*
>
> *Our system, if followed faithfully, will more or less do away with the need for taking these drugs. It will save you the time you spend going to and from the doctor's office. It will give you peace of mind.*

THE ONLY DRUGS that I have taken in the last 10 years are air-sick preventives like Marazine and Dramamine. Of the two I believe Dramamine is the least harmful. Outside of this I do not have need for drugs. Due to my healthy habits I no longer get headaches, nor do I get viruses or other sicknesses. *You* can accomplish the same thing, without drugs. Follow the *Prevention* system, take your vitamins, eat right, do calisthenics, walk an hour a day and soon you, too, will not need any drug crutches! But if you continue to be careless of your health, and have to take drugs to "palliate" conditions of sickness, then you won't get your mental apparatus into the keenest condition.

Cortisone is a typical drug known to affect the mind. One doctor attributed the suicide of one of his patients to cortisone. Another says that, in general, within a few hours after cortisone therapy, the patient experiences a feeling of irritability, restlessness, tension, or emotional instability.

The thing to do is *not* to get the conditions that call for the taking of cortisone. It is remarkable that the nutrition we have described to give mental health will also give general physical health. They are both related to each other—a healthy mind in a healthy body.

Digitalis Can Affect the Mind

Take the drug *digitalis*. It is an old standby that most doctors think of as completely harmless. They often prescribe a maintenance dose that isn't changed for years. Arnold S. Moe, M.D., writing in the *Illinois State Medical Journal* (June 9, 1959), remarks on a *Texas Medical Journal* account of 100 cases of digitalis poisoning. It was found that 12 milligrams of digitalis, taken as a daily maintenance dose, proved to be toxic. Of the 100 patients, 27 died and seven of these deaths were attributed directly to digitalis.

Dr. Moe tells of a 60-year-old patient who told his physician he was suffering from a "heart spell," characterized by rapid heartbeat. The doctor prescribed digitalis, and soon the poor fellow noticed that he could speak nothing but nonsense, sometimes for several days at a time, and could not control what he was saying! His eyes became irritated and played color tricks on him, yet there was no physiological disturbance of the eyes. The cause turned out to be the digitalis. Six days after discontinuing the drug, the man was completely normal.

I have had a heart condition since I have been eight years old. Twelve years ago I was turned down for life insurance because of it. I am keeping my heart in good action by the taking of large amounts of vitamin E, which aids the heart by good oxygenation. My whole system of nutrition and exercise enabled me a few years ago to take a five hour hike over a mountain, *with* my heart condition, and I have never taken any kind of medication for my heart.

I have also seen to it that two conditions have been maintained. I have reduced my blood pressure to normal without the use of drugs, and I have gotten my pulse down to normal by means of exercise.

Penicillin

Then there is penicillin. We know of the dangerous side effects of taking this drug, but few are aware that some of these effects are in the mental category. In an editorial in the *British Medical Journal*, May 21, 1960, it is stated that injections of procaine penicillin can be followed by mental disturbance. In one case, when a further dose was given, a psychotic episode recurred. These drugs in over-dosage have often produced cerebral disturbances.

Again in the *British Medical Journal*, Sept. 28, 1957, the drug *isoniazid* (used for tuberculosis) was discussed. The article states that peripheral neuropathy (nervous disease) and psychosis are both well-recognized side-effects which have not infrequently been encountered. The paper discussed five cases of psychosis in patients receiving isoniazid in normal dosage. Three of them responded completely to treatment with vitamin B complex. So—don't get tuberculosis!

High Blood Pressure Drugs

In cases of high blood pressure the drugs of the *Rauwolfia-Reserpine* group have been extensively used, and have frequently led to mental disturbances. The following is an example, related in *Northwestern Medicine* (August, 1956).

A white, male executive, 59 years old, was given a general check-up on May 3, 1955. His blood pressure was found to be 200/130. *Rauwolfia* was started. The patient was seen at frequent intervals through 1955 and felt well. At times the blood pressure dropped as low as 138/82. Early in October 1955, he complained of anxiety over increased responsibilities which were proposed at his work. This anxiety rapidly increased despite a vacation and the use of meprobamate. By the latter part of October 1955 he was totally unable to leave his home by himself, was extremely blue and pessimistic in his outlook, could not relax, and seemed completely unable to help himself. The *Rauwolfia* was discontinued, and he was referred to a psychiatrist on November 1, 1955. Although electro-shock therapy was considered, it was deemed inexpedient because of osteoporosis of the dorsal spine. With constant psychiatric care he failed to show any marked degree of improvement until February 1956.

To my mind, the use of as powerful a drug as *Rauwolfia* to bring down high blood pressure is idiocy! High blood pressure can be brought down by four things—(a) a no salt diet, (b) a lot of exercise, (c) no smoking, and (d) the use of garlic pills. There is a terrific mass of medical evidence, done mostly in Europe and in South America, which shows how effective garlic pills are to reduce the blood pressure. So why use such dangerous drugs?

Side Effects

We have barely scratched the surface on the subject of drug usage as a cause of mental disease. Whole books have been published on the side-effects of drugs, and it becomes clearer with the passage of time that there is *no* drug that has no side-effect. In order for a drug to do its work it must be water-soluble. This means that it penetrates into every one of the billions of cells of the body. Drugs are used because they have overpowering effects in the situation that is giving trouble, but they also get into the blood circulation, and circulate into every nook and cranny, every tissue in the body, including the head, and into places where there is no trouble.

I recall that in 1935, when I published a little magazine called *Fact Digest,* I gave a doctor an assignment for an article with the theme—"How do drugs and medicines know where to go in the body to accomplish their effects." He never came back with the article. I never knew why, but *now* I think I know. Drugs work by a sledge-hammer method. Like firemen at a fire, they batter their way to the fire, but do a lot of damage on the way.

Drugs Are Soluble, Thus Finding Their Way to Every Cell Fed by the Bloodstream

The best way to safeguard your mental health is to follow a program which not only will maintain your health, but also will improve it! Keep your body strong and your nutrition good. Follow the *Prevention* program! Health consciousness can easily be developed so that you will rarely have need of a doctor or of his drugs—not even aspirin!

Doctors are too quick with their drugs. I recall in Florida a few years ago when my wife suffered a strained ligament in her foot, the doctor wished to inject cortisone. I objected.

"It could cause a softening of the spine and affect the mind," I said.

"Not in this amount," he replied.

"My wife happens to be very healthy. Her powers of recuperating are great. She does not need any cortisone!"

And she didn't get it either. But when we were given the bill by his nurse, there was $5.00 there for cortisone, with the word "cortisone" printed on the bill. He evidently gave cortisone to practically all his cases, which must have added up to a tidy sum at the end of the year. The nurse was amazed when we told her we had not taken the cortisone.

It may not be possible for you to cut out drugs altogether, especially at the beginning, but do keep them down to a minimum. In the long run, after following our program, you will find that eventually your body will become so healthy that you won't need the help or effect of any drugs.

REVIEW

Plenty of meat, fish, and eggs.

Low starch consumption, but include potatoes rather than bread.

No sugar and salt.

No tobacco or alcohol.

Vitamin A and D halibut liver oil perles.

Vitamin B, wheat germ, brewer's yeast, desiccated liver.

Vitamin C, Rose hips.

Vitamin E, mixed tocopherols in good quantity.

Kelp tablets—for minerals.

Exercise—calisthenics and walks.

No refined foods.

No factory produced goods.

No drugs, especially no aspirins.

Favor foods that have been somewhat protected against poisons.

20

Chiropractic Treatments and the Nervous System

> *Perhaps you have never been to a chiropractor. Perhaps you are afraid he will hurt you! I have never been hurt by a chiropractor and I have been going to them regularly on a health maintenance basis for the last 30 years or so! I always feel invigorated when I come out of their office.*
>
> *Their treatments are a stimulation to the nervous system and to the bloodstream. They are definitely good for you in helping you to use your brain to its maximum power.*

THE PUBLIC SHOULD be acquainted with the fact that chiropractic treatment has a great deal to offer not only to a mental patient, but also to people who are not up to par in the ability to use their brain. There is a definite type of spinal distortion to be found in mental cases. A correction of such distortion may result in an improvement or a complete correction of mental illness.

What I have written is based on an article by Dr. D. B. Mears, a chiropractor, in the March 1964 issue of *Prevention.*

I will quote Dr. Mears:

WHAT X-RAY SHOWS

The basis of the author's research rests upon the study of over ten thousand X-rays taken from a lateral aspect of the head and the neck area of the spine. In order to determine the abnormal, it was first necessary to establish the range of normality as regards the lateral X-ray of the cervical (neck) spine and head. By the use of certain relative anatomical lines and the study of many X-rays, a range of normality depending on the relative position of the head and spine was established.

Let us assume that the normal patient has an accident. Perhaps he falls and hits the back of his head, or he may hit the forward part of his head on top of a car while his head is tipped forward, or he may receive a jolt which snaps his head forward. There are many possible accidents that may occur, some of which might occur at birth. Many seem so trivial that they are completely forgotten. Later, however, the patient is aware that he is becoming nervous. An X-ray gives obvious evidence that the patient's accident has tipped the head forward and downward. The extension of distance creates a pulling tension on the spinal cord and brain and the patient is fully aware that something is amiss, even though he may not recall the accident. Patients with such distortions fall in the category of the neurotic and those with thyroid involvement. Seldom are they psychotic. After an adjustment is given to restore the widened distance to normal, the patient often remarks: "What a relief. I feel alive again. The adjustment felt like the opening of a faucet."

It is sometimes possible to detect this type of distortion even before the X-ray is taken. Perhaps the reader has noticed a person who occasionally tips his head well back and then shakes it from side to side. This is a subconscious desire to restore the head-spine relationship to normal.

MILLIONS NEED CHIROPRACTIC

There are probably millions of nervous patients in this nation who have this type of distortion. The greatest percentage of these people, due to medical propaganda, do not consult a chiropractor, and their case likely progresses from Stage One to Stage Two. In Stage One the gravitational force is at a point too far forward in the head, which results from a forward tipping of the head. This unbalanced pull of gravity exerts itself at all times when the patient is in a sitting or standing position. Eventually it leads to the Second Stage.

In this Stage, the pull of gravity has drawn the head and the entire neck region of the spine to a much more forward position. The patient is now more nervous and depressed and he may be in the psychotic episode stage. His friends will likely say to him: "Buck up, old boy! Look not down but up." Needless to say, with this type of distortion, this is easier said than done. Perhaps some brave friend of the patient suggests consulting a chiropractor but the chances are that the family opposes the idea, and, of course, the patient is by now in such a state of mental confusion that logical thinking is out of the question. And so, with few exceptions, the patient passes on into Stage Three and is "taken away."

This Third Stage of postural defect will be noticed by anyone who visits a mental institution. Even the psychiatrist has noticed the stooped posture of the mental patient, with the outjutting chin. Believe it or not, his explanation is that the mental patient is attempting to again assume the embryonic position as found in the womb. He is convinced that the disease has produced the postural defect. It never occurs to him that the postural defect has caused the disease.

X-ray examination reveals the vast difference that exists between a normally balanced spine and the X-ray findings of the psychotic patient. Even to the casual observer it becomes obvious that the posture of the psychotic is far from normal.

LARGE SCALE INVESTIGATION

In 1950 the author decided that his X-ray findings needed verification in Chiropractic mental institutions. In Davenport, Iowa, there are two such mental sanatoriums: The Clear View Sanatorium and the Forest Park Sanatorium. The X-ray studies conducted in these sanatoriums established the fact that there is, beyond doubt, a definite postural defect to be found in mental disease. In one institution it was found that 94 percent of the patients had these spinal distortions, and in the second institution 100 percent of the patients were so afflicted.

By the study of X-rays alone, and without seeing the patient, it was possible to determine the severity of the mental condition. By a study of X-rays, before and after Chiropractic care, it was possible to tell whether the patient's condition was improved, worse, or remained the same. This, I think, any unbiased person would agree, falls in the realm of science.

Dr. William Coulter, Research Director of the International Chiropractic Association, aided the author in the tabulation of the findings in these two mental institutions. In fact Doctor Coulter, by bringing into play his statistical aptitude, was able to predict, within a six-month period, the duration of the mental condition in eighteen out of twenty cases. This was done by figuring the severity of the spinal distortion according to the degree of change shown on the X-ray. Of the two cases that Doctor Coulter failed to calibrate correctly, it was found that one suffered from senile dementia and the second case was of severe traumatic origin with mental symptoms developing within a few hours after the accident. In this second case the injury to the patient had been so severe that Stage Three was created at the moment of the accident. Doctor Coulter's tabulations are another proof that certain spinal distortions are definitely a causative factor in the production of mental disease.

The writer goes to a chiropractor once a week, and whether you need it or not I would suggest that you do likewise; go at least twice a month. It is a form of insurance. It will aid you in maintaining the correct mechanical condition of your spine, and the health of your nervous system. If there is anything wrong in these two categories which stem from a mechanical distortion, then no amount of nutrition will give you the maximum of your mental power.

21

Natural Health and
the Divorce Rate

> This chapter is more ammunition in my scheme
> of getting you to embrace the program outlined
> in this book. It might save your marriage from
> going on the rocks. If you are married, have your
> marital partner read this book, especially if you
> both tend to bicker about small things that lead up
> to violent arguments.
>
> Wouldn't it be strange if too much ice-cream
> and cokes are endangering your marriage!

YOU MIGHT ASK, why waste space about divorce? What has
divorce got to do with a system to produce more mental
and physical energy? I will answer by saying that this same
system may improve your character. This same system
may save your marriage, may make you a better father,
mother, sister, or brother! Do you object to that? I merely
want to show you that divorce, as a rule, is an expression
of failure, of a lack of intelligence, or perhaps even an
example of ignorance, stupidity, or other negative charac-
teristics.

I would also like to maintain that a person in full
possession of a hard-hitting mentality, who is not mentally
sluggish or lazy, will see enough beforehand to break up a

courtship that does not have a chance of making the grade into a permanent marriage. I maintain that many pre-married couples who know that something is wrong, don't have enough mental energy to face up to the facts and break it off.

Thus, the rate of divorce is becoming appalling. In California today, for example, one out of two marriages is sure to hit the rocks, with a terrible disruption in the lives of the residual children, and affecting many others disastrously. In the nation generally, one out of four will be divorced.

A Doctor's Experience

Cecelia Rosenfeld, M.D. of Los Angeles, had an idea that many of her patients who were at the point of divorce, were that way because they had become emotional "cases" on account of poor nutrition. She began to work on these "cases" with a great deal of success, and wrote about it in a medical journal called *New Medical Materia* (August, 1962). I will reproduce her article herewith:

NUTRITIONAL GUIDANCE CAN FORESTALL BROKEN MARRIAGES

By Cecelia Rosenfeld, M.D.

Broken marriages have many causes. When quarreling couples appear before a psychiatrist or marriage counselor, they are duly encouraged to discuss their emotional, psychological, and sexual problems.

However, one of the prime causes of marital discord—nutritional deficiency—is too often over-looked.

In my own practice, I have found that a surprising number of "broken marriage" spouses suffered from a blood-sugar imbalance. Many of these husbands and wives showed symptoms of irritability, violent temper, abnormal sensitivity, and extreme fatigue. In most cases, there was no evidence of organic disease.

Corrective nutritional guidance dispelled these unpleasant symptoms for many spouses, and in the process often bolstered their crumbling marriages.

Of course, nutritional deficiencies are not confined to married persons. Bachelors, spinsters, children—anyone—can become physically and emotionally ill because of poor nutrition. But it is in the marriage situation, where the emotional outlook of husband and wife are so intimately connected, that truculence and short temper most often "rub the wrong way."

As these symptoms seem to indicate a need for investigation in the area of *hypoglycemia* (low blood sugar), a four-hour glucose tolerance test is usually recommended.

The glucose tolerance tests generally reveal a pattern of abnormal fluctuations in the glucose (sugar) levels. Of greatest significance is the relatively precipitous drop in the glucose level.

The symptoms are most pronounced at the low point. It is not so much the level as the rapid rate of the drop within the test period. The glucose curve often points up which gland is involved in the endocrine imbalances.

Briefly, it may be concluded that many of these symptoms have their origin in a metabolic imbalance. This imbalance, in turn, may be caused by ingestion of excessive amounts of carbohydrates or alcohol.

A sugar imbalance may cause emotional stress. On the other hand, emotional stress may cause a sugar imbalance.

Whatever the initial cause of the disturbance, patients showing such nutritional deficiency should be placed on a corrective diet. The essential features of this diet are low carbohydrate ingestion and emphasis on proteins and fats.

They should be instructed to omit sugar in all forms—soft drinks, pastry, ice cream, or the like. In most instances, patients should be advised to eat six light meals per day in order to maintain a stable glucose level. Vegetables and fruit provide sufficient carbohydrates to maintain nutritional balance.

Within a few weeks after starting on their new diet, an impressive majority of my "broken marriage" patients showed a positive response. Here are two typical examples:

Case No. 1

Case 1: Mrs. R.L., a 34-year-old secretary, was referred to me by a psychoanalyst. Her symptoms included exhaustion, fatigue, exceedingly poor concentration, and chronic depression. As a result of these symptoms, her home life had deteriorated and she was separated from her husband.

Mrs. R.L. had been taking two grains of thyroid daily for a number of years. After six weeks on a nutritional regimen, the thyroid dosage was reduced to one grain, and eventually reduced even further.

Four months later, improvement was so marked that Mrs. R.L. resumed post-graduate work which had been discontinued because of her condition. She is living with her husband again, and both report that the marriage situation is harmonious.

Case No. 2

Case 2: Mr. T.E., a 53-year-old business executive, was referred by a marriage counseling service. He had been suffering from severe migraine headaches for ten years—especially severe during the night. During these years, the patient had been treated at two major clinics and under private care. According to Mr. T.E.: "Every night, I swallowed an assortment of pills to ease the pain."

Mr. T.E.'s wife had complained that his chronic irritability made him impossible to live with—she had begun divorce proceedings.

The patient was advised to discontinue all medication, and was given a nutritional program instead. In two months, the headaches had disappeared.

Mr. T.E. and his wife have since taken a six-month trip around the world. His wife's statement at the conclusion of treatment was: "He has become an energetic companion and a good husband."

My work in nutrition began 14 years ago and grew out of my experience common to all

NATURAL HEALTH AND THE DIVORCE RATE 145

ophthalmologists, in observing certain systemic disease through eye-examinations.

At that time, there were few medical practitioners specializing in nutritional guidance, and I felt an obligation to pursue studies in bio-chemistry and endocrinology.

When I applied these studies to my practice, I found that not only eye conditions were improved—patients also reported conditions in such conditions as hypertension, heart ailments, gastro-intestinal dysfunctions, and obesity.

One of the most gratifying concomitant benefits of nutritional guidance is that, in alcoholics, the craving for liquor often diminishes.

Case No. 3

For example, Mrs. L.T., a 28-year-old housewife, was referred to me by a psychoanalyst with the information that alcoholism might be the basis for her marriage troubles. Both Mrs. L.T. and her husband were described as basically intelligent and responsible individuals.

The patient apparently was a victim of the so-called "obligations" of her social circle, which included much drinking of hard liquor.

Mrs. L.T.'s condition when intoxicated was severely affecting her husband's business and social relationships. The husband also reported that their two young children were exhibiting intense negative reactions to the situation.

After five weeks of nutritional guidance, the patient reported that she felt wonderful and was able to resume her domestic responsibilities. Except for occasional lapses, the patient now restricts herself to one glass of wine per day.

Unlike other therapies which are directed primarily to the relief of specific conditions, nutritional guidance is a form of preventive medicine. When a person achieves sound nutritional habits, he gains a lifelong pattern for healthful living.

Dr. Rosenfeld has asked us to stress that marital problems are not her primary field of practice. Her main interest is nutritional guidance of children to prevent future emotional and degenerative disease problems.

Before leaving this chapter, I would like to mention that, a few years ago, the U.S. Public Health Service made a grant of $33,101, described as follows:

"A test of the husband-wife relationship. The aim is to develop a diagnostic pictorial test of both intrapersonal and interpersonal aspects of the role relationship of husband and wife. The test should be sensitive to the perceptions of actual behavior and norms and to the consonance perceived between these."

I am not making any comment!

22

The Amazing Results of the Rodale System

AGNES Z. TLUSTUS of 173¼ Douglas Street, Los Angeles, who has practiced the *Prevention* system for many years, recently wrote me, "When I passed the bar examination last March, I was astonished. They are so difficult! I understand that only three out of every 10 pass, and I was the only girl among the men!" I know how she feels because I have seen a gradual improvement in my own mental ability. And I know how you will feel, five or six months after you start on this system. Nothing like it has ever been tried before and I can guarantee the results in 99 out of 100 cases.

Here is a letter from an 82-year-old lady reader of *Prevention*, Mrs. Lee J. Smith, Hotel Faber, Mendota, Illinois . . . "So many friends are laid low with what we used to consider the common cold. I haven't had a cold for five or six years! I go out every morning—unless too much ice is on the streets—often with my coat open at the neck, but since reading *Prevention* I add many supplements to my diet—bone meal, wheat germ, brewer's yeast, etc. I am happier than so many younger persons I meet who are always complaining and having a battle with living, and the problems they must meet."

Happiness is part of the achievement that can be obtained from following the system outlined in this book —also a graceful, non-senile old age with the mind young and controlled.

It is all a matter of putting these things into practice— getting into the habit. It will soon become so ingrained that it will no longer be a chore. Thousands of readers of

Prevention have testified to it. It is not that I'm trying to sell you a fake gold mine or some blue sky. If what I say is not true, why would I, a successful businessman, recommend it? It would only hit back into my face and make me a figure of ridicule! Can I afford to take that chance?

So what do you have to lose? Only money! And how much money have you frittered away on really "wild-goose" ideas? I offer you an investment with assured returns—an investment of cash, with the returns in a far more valuable medium of exchange.

Put this method into practice, and in the end it will be money in your pocket because, when your general mental ability has improved, you will earn more in many ways—a better job, a better investment policy for your personal monies, a better ability to conserve your financial resources, and prevention of possible divorce or of an automobile accident! They all add up to money saved.

If you are a heavy smoker, you might find it difficult to stop smoking, but I will venture that if you take the rest of the plan, and leave the smoking cure for the last, it will come easier at that time. I am sure that in six months or so you will find yourself a different person.

In my own case I have found that the system keeps working progressively; it will produce results for you for a great many years. What I mean is that at the end of two weeks or so I felt slightly better—I call this the two week effect. Two months later I felt still better. This is the two months effect. Then there are the one year, two year, and three year effects—always an improvement, because the good nutrition is slowly repairing all your nerves, glands, and organs, and all this takes time.

I have been on the system about 14 years and can still feel mental and physical improvements. Right now I am on the 14 year effect. My ability to write plays is greatly improving, and I am able to keep direct contact with my eight or nine projects, as well as continually starting new ones. I am only 67. But you just wait till I'm 86. What fun to look forward to, with never a let-up to a spirit of creativity. After all, there were old people who accomplished great things—Titian, the artist, Ben Franklin, the essayist, John Quincy Adams, the statesman, and many others. But they were nourished with more potent food, food grown in non-chemicalized soils, and not tampered with in the food factories.

Now I would like to say a few words from a surprising

angle. To be a part of raising the general level of intelligence of the U.S. is nothing less than patriotism! You might say "I'm plenty smart enough for my britches." Yes! But don't forget that life today is different. Only a few years ago, there would come an occasional war and the soldiers would go off to some front. But today the front is right here in our midst. We are all soldiers! There may never be another "front" war. In the future they will be shooting at all of us right in our homes, if they ever shoot.

So, it is part of our duty to our country to develop the whole level of our intelligence, so as to be able to handle our personal, political, and business lives in such a way that we can maintain our independence, while living in peace with the rest of the world.

In such a program Russia is far ahead of us. When my son shot with the champion U.S. Skeet team at Cairo a few years ago, he noticed that the Russians brought their own food along! The Russians permit far less chemicalization of their factory-made food. Evidently the Russians believe that by good nutrition the mind can function better, and that their shooters could shoot straighter, for it is the mind that influences the gun. My son helped the Americans beat the Russians. On the American team he made the highest score, and he was the only civilian—the other three were soldiers! He is a product of a very high quality nutrition.

Russia is getting ahead of us in the health of its citizens. Note that the Russian mortality figures are going down. Ours are going up, and our birth rate has been going down for the last two years.

The Russians use far less tobacco per capita than we do, far less soft drinks, candy and such. They also permit far less artificial coloring of foods with coal tar chemicals. If there is a race for world supremacy, and if brain power is to enter into it, Russia is already far ahead of us.

Patriotism is a peculiar thing. It seems to consist of a flag gathering dust in some closet, and when a war comes along, we take it out and wave it! Well, my friends, things are going to be different from now on. Patriotism is now—at your dinner table! By our nation eating itself into a better mentality, we can save money in less crime, less hospitals, more schools and better pay for teachers, and more money to build a strong defense against the communist world!

So get going, and let's make the U.S. physically and mentally the keenest nation in all the world!

Index